Table of Contents

Preface

Reports of the Council on Ethical and Judicial Affairs

The Council on Ethical and Judicial Affairs is composed of nine members, eight physicians and one medical student. All are members of the American Medical Association. Each is nominated by the President of the AMA and elected by the House of Delegates, the AMA's representative assembly. Council members are selected on the basis of their distinguished accomplishments in medicine, their professional compassion and integrity, and their commitment to establishing ethical standards for the medical profession.

The AMA's Code of Medical Ethics is composed of four parts. The *Principles of Medical Ethics* are seven precepts that broadly define the parameters of ethical conduct for physicians. *Fundamental Elements of the Patient-Physician Relationship* enunciates the basic rights to which patients are entitled from their physicians. *Current Opinions* is a comprehensive set of concise statements addressing specific ethical issues in the practice of medicine. *Current Opinions* with Annotations includes, in addition to these statements, summaries of court rulings and the medical and legal literature that cite to specific Opinions.

Finally, the Council Reports contain scholarly analyses of current issues in medical ethics. Comprehensive and extensively referenced, these Reports provide the reasoning that led to many of the Opinions found in *Current Opinions*. The Reports are issued twice yearly, after the Annual and Interim meetings of the AMA's House of Delegates. The subjects of the Reports are chosen for their relevance to contemporary bioethical thought and ethical dilemmas arising in the practice of medicine. The constant issuance of new Reports, and Opinions based upon them, assures that the AMA's Code of Medical Ethics is always a live document and always a work-in-progress.

All four components of the AMA's Code of Medical Ethics need to be consulted to determine the Association's positions on ethical issues. In addition, the AMA's House of Delegates at times issues statements on ethical issues. These statements are contained in a separate publication, the *AMA Policy Compendium*. Because the Council on Ethical and Judicial Affairs is responsible for determining the AMA's positions on ethical issues, statements by the House of Delegates should be construed as the view of the House of Delegates and not as the ethics policy of the Association.

Introduction to This Compendium

This compendium is a compilation of Council Reports from 1990 to 1997 that examine a variety of ethical issues that have arisen in the era of managed care. These Reports are published here in a form substantially unchanged from that in which they were originally adopted. The only exceptions are those Reports that have been revised slightly and published in the medical literature since their issuance. For those, the published rather than the originally adopted version is supplied. The content of earlier Reports may be superseded by that of later Reports – in particular, some terms and

American Medical Association

Physicians dedicated to the health of America

Council on Ethical and Judicial Affairs

Reports on Managed Care

Council on Ethical and Judicial Affairs Reports on Managed Care

Internet address: http://www.ama-assn.org

Additional copies (product number OP049898) may be ordered from:

Order Department
American Medical Association
515 North State Street
Chicago, IL 60610
800 621-8355

ISBN 0-89970-963-X

BP25:98-666:1.5M:8/98

statistics may be dated. In those areas where significant discrepancy exists between old and new Reports, an endnote has been inserted referring the reader to the most current position of the Council.

The Council hopes that this compendium will serve as a valuable resource and educational tool for those wishing to understand the ethical challenges posed by managed care.

June 1998.

Council on Ethical and Judicial Affairs 1997-1998

Robert M. Tenery, Jr, MD, Chair
Herbert Rakatanksy, MD, Vice Chair
Alan Hartford, MD, PhD
John C. Madden, III
Leonard J. Morse, MD
John M. O'Bannon, III, MD
Frank A. Riddick, Jr, MD
Victoria N. Ruff, MD
George T. Wilkins, Jr, MD

Linda L. Emanuel, MD, PhD, Vice President, Ethics Standards
Stephen R. Latham, JD, PhD, Council Secretary
H. Nina Kim, Staff Associate
Blaire S. Osgood, Staff Associate

Financial Incentives to Limit Care: Financial Implications for HMOs and IPAs

Resolution 28 (I-88), which was referred to the Board of Trustees, requests a study "to provide an updated description of standards for the receiving of fees for services from all payors... in the context of health maintenance organizations (HMOs), independent practice associations (IPAs), and joint ventures."

The Council on Ethical and Judicial Affairs recommends the adoption of the following report in lieu of Resolution 28 (I-88).

Overview

The physician-patient relationship is built on a foundation of mutual trust. It is the confidence inspired by this relationship that enables patients to place their health and well-being in the hands of physicians. At least since the time of Hippocrates, physicians have cultivated the trust of their patients by professing to place patient welfare before all other concerns. This tradition of placing primary emphasis on the interests of the patient has endured through the ages as the guiding tenet of medical practice.

In recent years, however, pressures to contain spiraling health care costs have tended to create a potential for conflict between the interests of patients and physicians. Patients in America have come to expect access to the best available care, regardless of its costs. They trust their physicians to do all that is possible to enhance their health and well-being. Physicians, however, increasingly have conflicting obligations to their patients and to those who finance medical services. Not only are physicians expected to serve as advocates for their patients in obtaining appropriate diagnostic and therapeutic services, but they also are expected, in their relationships with third-party payors, to contain health care expenditures. This conflict is evident, for example, when the remuneration received by physicians is tied, through the use of financial inducements, to the degree of cost containment achieved in the provision of medical services.

Conflicts of Interest in Health Care Delivery Systems

Potential economic conflicts of interest are inherent to the practice of medicine. Health care services traditionally have been rendered on a fee-for-service basis, whereby physicians receive compensation for each diagnostic or therapeutic service provided to a patient. In such a setting, an incentive exists to increase the number of services rendered. These potential conflicts of interest, which are beyond the scope of this report, have been addressed in a more comprehensive manner in a separate Board of Trustees report.

Alternative practice settings also are characterized by potential conflicts between the interests of physicians and patients. Managed care plans that include, for example, HMOs and IPAs may provide physicians with economic incentives to limit the medical services provided to patients. Increasingly, these incentives include direct financial rewards for physicians who help the organization to achieve their cost-containment objectives. The nature of these rewards may vary with the organizational structure and compensation practices of the managed health care plan.

The Organizational Structure of HMOs and IPAs

The organizational structure of HMOs differs from that of fee-for-service systems in the methods used to compensate physicians and in the general degree of emphasis on cost containment. HMOs typically agree to provide all necessary medical services to an enrolled population in return for a fixed premium, paid on a monthly or yearly basis. In theory, HMOs are able to reduce health care expenditures in at least two important respects.

First, HMOs promote cost savings by encouraging early, office-based treatment. The presumption here is that routine, preventive care is cost-efficient, whereas treatment of acute conditions that, because of financial concerns, have been left unattended ultimately may require more costly intervention or hospitalization.

Second, some HMOs limit their costs by placing institutional controls on patient access to costly services, such as hospitalization or referrals to medical specialists. For example, patients often must obtain prior authorization from an HMO primary care physician before consulting a medical specialist. Failure to do so may result in the HMO's refusal to provide reimbursement for the unauthorized care. Medical referrals may be further restricted to a particular physician, group, or facility that is responsive to the cost containment objectives of the HMO. These restrictions customarily are conveyed to potential members of the HMO prior to enrollment, and therefore represent voluntary conditions of participation.

With increasing frequency, some HMOs attempt to achieve additional savings by providing participating physicians with a variety of financial incentives to contain the overall costs of the medical services provided to their patients. The structure and effectiveness of these inducements tends to vary with the organizational characteristics of the HMO and with the methods used by the organization to compensate participating physicians.

Four organizational models of HMOs have been described: (1) the staff model, in which health care services are delivered to an enrolled population through employed physicians responsible directly to the health maintenance organization; (2) the group model, in which the HMO contracts with an independent group of physicians to provide medical services to qualified enrollees; (3) the network model, in which the HMO contracts with two or more group practices; and (4) the independent practice association (IPA) model, in which independent physicians contract with the HMO to provide comprehensive medical services to an assigned patient population.

HMOs also use variable structures to compensate physicians. The three arrangements commonly used for primary care physicians are: (1) salaries; (2) fee-for-service; and (3) capitation arrangements. Under fee-for-service compensation arrangements, HMOs base their payments to physicians on the actual charges incurred in the provision of particular services, the customary and prevailing charges in the physician's geographic area of practice, or a predetermined fee schedule. Capitation fees, on the other hand, provide participating physicians with a fixed monthly or yearly payment per HMO enrollee. The physician then is obligated to provide certain types of medical services (eg, primary care) to the enrolled population during the benefit period, regardless of cost. Capitation arrangements represent a form of financial risk sharing, whereby physicians profit only if the total costs of the medical services provided to enrollees is less than the sum of the capitation fees collected by the physician. If all clinically indicated care cannot be provided to the enrolled population for an amount that is less than or equal to the sum of the capitation fees, the physician may suffer a financial loss unless the HMO has sufficient reserves to cover the loss or some appropriate care is withheld.

Compensation arrangements in HMOs also may involve a variety of withholding schemes designed to shift a portion of the organization's financial risk to individual physicians. Typically, the premiums paid by enrollees are divided into a number of distinct accounts. The funds in each account are earmarked for specific types of expenses, such as administrative costs, primary care, referrals to specialists, hospitalization, and outpatient diagnostic tests.

A percentage of the revenue that is allocated to primary care accounts frequently is withheld from participating physicians until the end of the year to assure that adequate funds are available for referrals and other outside services. If, at the end of the year, an overall surplus exists in an account that is earmarked for a specific type of service, the withheld portion may be returned to the HMOs physicians. Surplus amounts above and beyond the initial withholding also may be distributed to participating physicians, either individually or as a group, as a bonus or reward for effective cost containment.

Similarly, the HMO may penalize physicians for year-end deficits in particular accounts by requiring them to forfeit the amounts withheld, or occasionally, by imposing additional financial penalties. The HMO may or may not place an upper limit on the extent of a physician's personal financial risk.

In the event of either a surplus or a deficit in the HMO's accounts, the corresponding bonus or penalty for physicians may be calculated individually, based on the total care provided by individual practitioners, or as a group, with the total financial benefit or risk equally distributed among all physicians.

Potential Effects of Financial Incentives

The use of financial incentives to promote cost awareness among HMO physicians has created some concern that such inducements could result in inappropriate reductions in the services made available to HMO patients. As noted in a 1988 GAO study:

> A primary purpose of HMO physician incentive plans is to get the physician to consider the cost implications of alternative courses for diagnosing or treating patients. The goal of such plans should be to encourage physicians to select the least expensive course of care that meets the patient's needs and results in adequate care. However, incentive plans may offer such strong financial incentives to physicians to reduce utilization that quality of care could be adversely effected through the withholding of needed services.[4]

This same study identified four characteristics of financial incentive plans that seem to have the greatest potential to adversely affect the quality of the medical services provided to HMO patients. The characteristics identified were: (1) the amount of financial risk that is shifted from the HMO to individual physicians; (2) the number of physicians whose performance is used to calculate monetary distributions; (3) whether the incentive payments are based on a percentage of individual provider savings or profits; and (4) the length of time over which the cost performance of physicians is measured. It was found, for example, that when performance is measured over a short period of time (eg, one month) such that incentive payments are closely linked to individual treatment decisions, financial inducements exert a greater influence on physician behavior.

The Impact of Financial Incentive Plan on Quality of Care

It is difficult to measure the impact of financial incentive programs on the quality and appropriateness of the care that is rendered to HMO participants.

Several studies have attempted to determine how HMOs achieve their cost savings. The results from these studies are not conclusive, nor are they consistent.

One study presented comparative data for eight discretionary procedures (eg, hysterectomies).[5] The findings revealed that HMOs do not differentially reduce discretionary procedures in order to achieve cost savings. In other words, according to this study, HMOs appear to contain medical costs by eliminating both discretionary and nondiscretionary inpatient procedures. Other studies also have found that fewer hospital admissions among HMO patients do not appear to result exclusively from reductions in those procedures that are viewed as discretionary.[6] However, a study of diagnostic testing practices among physicians did suggest that fewer discretionary outpatient tests are ordered for HMO enrollees than fee-for-service patients.

Ethical Considerations Involving Financial Incentive Plans

The primary responsibility of the medical profession is to benefit patients. Physicians have an ethical obligation to place the health and well-being of their patients before all other concerns. If a conflict develops between physicians' personal financial interests and their obligations to a patient, the physician must not permit the patient's health and well-being to be compromised.

Financial inducements must not be permitted to taint a physician's judgment of appropriate therapeutic alternatives. Such alternatives should be disclosed to the patient, who then is at liberty to make an informed decision about his or her medical treatment, based upon the information provided. It would be unethical for a physician to deny his or her patients access to appropriate medical services based upon the promise of personal financial reward.

If the treatment alternatives available to a patient are limited by contractual agreement, such limitations should be fully disclosed, as noted in Opinion 8.13 of *Current Opinions of the Council on Ethical and Judicial Affairs of the American Medical Association*, 1989:

> **Referral of Patients/Disclosure of Limitations.** When a physician agrees to provide treatment, he thereby enters into a contractual relationship and assumes an ethical obligation to treat the patient to the best of his ability. PPO and HMO contracts generally restrict the participating physician's scope of referral to medical specialists, diagnostic laboratories, and hospitals that have contractual arrangements with the PPO or HMO. Some plans also restrict the circumstances under which referrals may be made to contracting medical specialists. If the PPO or HMO does not permit referral to a noncontracting medical specialist or to a diagnostic or treatment facility when the physician believes that the patient's condition requires such services, the physician should so inform the patient so that the patient may decide whether to accept the outside referral at his own expense or confine himself to services available within the PPO or HMO. In determining whether treatment or diagnosis requires referral to outside specialty services, the physician should be guided by standards of good medical practice.

As suggested by tradition, patient welfare must be the primary concern of physicians. The Council on Ethical and Judicial Affairs therefore recommends adoption of the following statement to address the potentially adverse effects of financial inducements on the quality and appropriateness of patient care:

1. Physicians must not deny their patients access to appropriate medical services based upon the promise of personal financial reward, or the avoidance of financial penalties.

2. Patients must have the necessary information to make informed decisions about their care. Physicians therefore have an ethical obligation to assure the disclosure of medically appropriate treatment alternatives, regardless of cost.

3. Physicians must assure that their contractual agreements restricting referral or treatment options are disclosed to patients.

4. Physicians must assure disclosure of any financial inducements that may tend to limit the diagnostic and therapeutic alternatives that are offered to patients or that may tend to limit patients' overall access to care.

5. Physicians may satisfy their disclosure obligations by assuring that the managed care plan makes adequate disclosure to patients enrolled in the plan.

6. Physicians should promote an effective program of peer review to monitor and evaluate the quality and appropriateness of the patient care services provided within their practice setting.

Report of the Council on Ethical and Judicial Affairs of the American Medical Association.
June 1990.

Endnotes

1. InterStudy. *A Mid-Year Report on HMO Growth.* June 1986. Excelsior, Minn. InterStudy.

2. Hillman A, et al. How do financial incentives affect physicians' clinical decisions and the financial performance of health maintenance organizations? *N Engl J Med.* 1989;321:86-92.

3. Hillman A. Financial incentives for physicians in HMO's: Is there a conflict of interest? *N Engl J Med.* 1987;1743-1748.

4. GAO: Medicare. *Physician Incentive Payments by Prepaid Health Plans Could Lower Quality of Care.* Report to the Chairman, Subcommittee on Health, Committee on Ways and Means. U.S. House of Representatives. December 1988.

5. Luft H. How do health maintenance organizations achieve their "savings"? Rhetoric and evidence. *N Engl J Med.* 1978;298:1336-1343.

6. Siu A. Inappropriate use of hospitals in a randomized trial of health insurance plans. *N Engl J Med.* 1986;315:1259-1266.

Ethical Issues in Managed Care

A primary concern of medical ethicists for some time has been the absence of any meaningful analysis of the impact of health care delivery marketplace changes and current legislative reforms on the essential tenets of the patient-physician relationship. Although President Clinton's original reform proposal addressed in broad terms the ethical imperatives supporting universal access, it left virtually unexamined the more fundamental question of the role of the physician in a reformed system in which the incentives are dramatically changed and budgets determine the amount of health care spending and services.

In June 1990, the Council on Ethical and Judicial Affairs issued a report, "Financial Incentives to Limit Care: Financial Implications for HMOs and IPAs,"[1] which described the financial incentives that managed care plans offer physicians to limit their provision of care. The report concluded that patient welfare must remain the first concern of physicians working in health maintenance organizations (HMOs) and independent practice associations (IPAs), and that physicians must disclose all relevant financial inducements and contractual restrictions that affect the delivery of health care to patients.

With its emphasis on managed care and managed competition, health system reform will greatly increase the salience of the ethical concerns raised by managed care. It is therefore essential that the profession and society act now to ensure that managed care techniques are implemented in a way that protects patients and the integrity of the patient-physician relationship.

In this report, the Council reiterates the physician's commitment to patient welfare first and updates its previous recommendations for physicians. This report discusses in greater detail the potential conflicts of interest faced by physicians practicing in the managed care environment. It then recommends measures to preserve the fundamental duty of physicians as patient advocates by reducing the risk of rationing and inappropriate financial incentives.

Background

As health care costs have risen and calls for more cost-conscious health care have been made,[2] health care insurers increasingly have adopted principles of managed care.[3] Several different types of managed care arrangements have gained prominence in the American health care system, including group- and staff-model HMOs, IPAs, and preferred provider organizations. Fee-for-service plans are also using many of the cost-saving techniques of managed care.

Managed care plans use a number of techniques. Some of them are directed at physician behavior. Others are directed at subscribers to the plan.[4,5] For example, managed care plans typically encourage subscribers to seek health care when it is still possible to prevent the development of illness by covering a broad range of preventive and primary care services.

In addition, they restrict subscribers to panels of physicians who have agreed to accept lower reimbursements or who may have exhibited a history of practicing lower-cost care. Managed care plans can also control their subscribers' behavior by denying access to the services of medical specialists until the subscriber has obtained the approval of a primary care physician.

Managed care plans constrain the costs of participating physician practices in several ways as well. The plans may restrict the ability of physicians to perform certain procedures or to order certain medications or diagnostic tests. For example, a physician may need the approval of a radiologist before ordering a diagnostic imaging test, or a managed care plan might exclude some expensive drugs from the plan's formulary. Managed care plans aggressively use programs of utilization review to detect what they consider medically inappropriate or unnecessarily costly practice patterns.

Managed care plans can also reduce costs by creating economies of scale by coordinating care among physicians and hospitals, by mandating the use of guidelines or parameters of care (*Chicago Tribune*. November 10, 1993:A1), and by establishing advanced information systems that provide an improved basis on which to measure quality and efficiency.

Managed care plans also encourage physicians to make cost-conscious treatment decisions through the use of financial incentives. The plans often compensate physicians with capitation fees or a salary. In addition, plans typically use incentives for physicians to limit their use of diagnostic tests, referrals to other physicians, hospital care, or other ancillary services. For example, managed care plans often pay bonuses to physicians, with the amount of the bonus increasing as the plans' expenditures for patient care decrease. Or plans often withhold a fixed percentage of their physicians' compensation until the end of the year to cover any shortfalls in the funds budgeted for expenditures on patient care. If there is no shortfall, or the shortfall can be covered by part of the withheld fees, the remaining withheld fees are returned to the physicians.[1]

While efforts to contain costs are critical, and while many of the approaches of managed care have an impact, managed care can compromise the quality and integrity of the patient-physician relationship and reduce the quality of care received by patients. In particular, by creating conflicting loyalties for the physician, some of the techniques of managed care can undermine the physician's fundamental obligation to serve as patient advocate. Moreover, in their zeal to control utilization, managed care plans may withhold appropriate diagnostic procedures or treatment modalities for patients. Indeed, the US Department of Health and Human Services recently expressed concerns about practices at a major HMO after receiving eight allegations of insufficient patient care (*Wall Street Journal*. October 3, 1994:A1).

The Patient-Physician Relationship

Before discussing the potential impact of managed care on the patient-physician relationship, it is important to consider what is at stake. The foundation of the patient-physician relationship is the trust that physicians are dedicated first and foremost to serving the needs of their patients. In the oath of Hippocrates, trust is a central element in almost all the ethical obligations of physicians: physicians must keep patients' private information confidential, avoid mischief and sexual misconduct, and give no harmful or death-causing agent. Patients can expect that physicians will come to their aid even if it means putting the physician's own health at risk,[6] and they can trust that physicians will do everything in their power to help their patients. It is this trust that enables patients to communicate private information and to place their health, and indeed their lives, in the hands of their physicians.[1] Without trust, the success of the healing process would be seriously diminished.

No other party in the health care system has the kind of responsibility that physicians have to advocate for patients, and no other party is in a position to assume that kind of responsibility. Physicians care for patients directly, are in the best position to know patients' interests, and can advocate within the health care system for patients' needs. Without the commitment that physicians place patients' interests first and act as agents for their patients alone, there is no assurance that the patient's health and well-being will be protected.

Ethical Concerns

Managed care involves at least two conflicting loyalties for the physician—conflicts that are not unique to managed care. First, physicians are expected to balance the interests of their patients with the interests of other patients. When deciding whether to order a test or procedure for a patient, the physician must consider whether the slot should be saved for another patient or not used at all to conserve the plan's resources. Second, managed care can place the needs of patients in conflict with the financial interests of their physicians. Managed care plans use bonuses and fee-withholds to make physicians cost conscious. As a result, when physicians are deciding whether to order a test, they will recognize that it may have an adverse impact on their income.

Some commentators argue that market forces will ensure that patients are protected from undue conflicts of interest. Because subscribers are theoretically free to choose their managed care organization based on quality of coverage, performance record, and other factors, they can theoretically drive those managed care organizations with the least impressive records out of business. However, it is unlikely that these consumer choices alone will ensure high-quality managed care organizations. As stated in a recent editorial, "patient satisfaction depends more on visible amenities and personal relations than on the quality and appropriateness of medical services..."[7]

The following two sections address the potential conflicts of interest for physicians under managed care.

Conflicts Among Patients

While some cost containment can be achieved by eliminating waste and inefficiency, it is also being achieved by limiting the availability of tests or procedures that offer only small or uncertain benefit or that provide a likely benefit but at a great expense. Because managed care plans generally work within a limited budget and, increasingly, are for-profit companies that compete to report favorable results to shareholders,[7,8] the cost of a service will influence whether the service is offered to patients who might benefit from it. Allocation rules are developed by the plans to deal with this issue.

Managed care plans can make these allocation decisions in a number of ways: by developing guidelines that determine for a physician when the service should be offered by instructing physicians to provide medically necessary care and delegating to the physicians the allocation decisions, or by some combination of allocation guidelines, physician discretion, and oversight.

An example of an allocation decision might involve the use of high-osmolar contrast media (HOCM) and low-osmolar contrast media (LOCM) in diagnostic imaging procedures.[9] Both HOCM and LOCM produce images of similar quality and are approved by the Food and Drug Administration as safe and effective. Adverse reactions, including "changes in cardiac performance, alterations in renal function, depression of the central nervous system, pain at the site of injection, flushing, nausea, and vomiting,"[9] are somewhat more likely with the use of HOCM. In addition, fatal adverse reactions with both media are extremely rare and no more likely with HOCM than LOCM.[10 (p616), 11] However there is a significant difference in the cost of the two media: LOCM are considerably more expensive than HOCM. Whereas a peripheral arteriography procedure would use about $10 worth of HOCM, the same procedure would use about $180 worth of LOCM, an increase of 18 times the HOCM cost.[9]

It is not obvious which contrast medium should be used. In fact, the decision to use HOCM or LOCM is essentially a value judgment about the relative costs and benefits of the two different media. While medical expertise is necessary to determine what benefits and risks are associated with the two media, the weighing of those benefits and risks with financial costs is not simply a medical decision but also a social judgment about the value of spending additional resources to lower health risks in this manner. A more difficult allocation case involves the use of bone marrow transplants for certain kinds of advanced cancer. The stakes for the patient are high—a prolonged life if successful—but the costs are great and the likelihood of success uncertain. Some plans will restrict or discourage the treatment; others may make it available under some circumstances.

Ethical Problems With Bedside Rationing

Physicians make cost-benefit judgments every day as a part of their professional responsibility in treating patients. It is unethical to knowingly provide unnecessary care or to be wasteful in providing needed care.

Allocation judgments about costs and services that approach a "rationing" decision—the denial of a procedure that benefits a patient—are not part of the physician's traditional role and, indeed, conflict with it. Although physicians have traditionally served as de facto gatekeepers to the health care system, overseeing the public's use of medical care, the cost-primacy environment of managed care significantly complicates this role.[13] As Pellegrino has written, "This [gatekeeper] role is morally dubious because it generates a conflict between the responsibilities of the physician as a primary advocate of the patient and as guardian of society's resources."[13] While this responsibility to guard society's resources is an important one, physicians must remain primarily dedicated to the health care needs of their individual patients.

The primary care physician's role in managed care illustrates the ethical problems associated with bedside rationing. The physician-gatekeeper determines whether the patient will be granted further access to the health care system, including referrals to specialists and diagnostic tests. At the same time, the physician is required by rules and encouraged by incentives to be aware of the overall financial limitations of the managed care entity for which he or she works.[4] The physician knows that there are other patients who have subscribed to the managed care plan and who are owed a certain level of health care.[14] These competing concerns mean that a patient's further treatment depends not only on the physician's judgment about the legitimacy of that patient's present medical need, but also on the relative weight of that need in comparison with the organization's need to serve all patients and control costs. Inconsistent and uninformed decisions are inevitable.

The primary care physician has the greatest responsibility within the managed care organization to assess the seriousness of patients' conditions accurately. A keen understanding of common and uncommon health problems is therefore required, as it is of all primary care physicians. However, the pressures of cost containment may encourage some physicians to try to manage cases longer than they should. Physicians may feel compelled to stretch their competence to keep patients at the primary care level and conserve resources. Inappropriate treatment and improper or missed diagnoses are potential outcomes of such decisions to delay or deny referral.

Preserving the Physician's Role

The physician is obligated to provide or recommend treatment when the physician believes that the treatment will materially benefit the patient and not to withhold the treatment to preserve the plan's resources. Physicians should not engage in bedside rationing.

But many allocation decisions are within arguable ranges or gray areas of at least minimally acceptable treatment. There are two steps to reducing patient-physician conflict in these circumstances. First, allocation decisions should be determined not by individual physicians at the bedside but according to guidelines established at a higher policymaking level. Physicians should contribute their expertise in the development of the guidelines and should advocate for the consideration of differences among patients. For example, it might be advisable for a certain group of patients at high risk to be offered LOCM while others who are not in this group are offered HOCM. Physicians can help ensure that all medically relevant information is considered and that no group of patients is put at an unfair disadvantage.

Second, and more importantly, even if the use of the LOCM were prohibited by a guideline for all or a particular class of patients, it remains the physician's duty to recommend its use and to advocate for the patient's right to the treatment in any case in which material benefit to a particular patient would result.

The structure through which physicians offer their expertise in policy-level decisions is very important. To help define this structure, the American Medical Association (AMA) recently proposed legislation[15] that would require managed care organizations to establish a medical staff structure, much like that in existence in every hospital in the United States. This proposal includes a governing board for the managed care organization that would include at least three physician members as representatives of participating physicians and a medical board composed entirely of participating physicians. Physicians on the medical board would be responsible for periodically reviewing restrictions on services to subscribers and other issues related to health care coverage. They would also review quality of care and physician credentialing on a periodic basis and disclose their review criteria to subscribers. The governing board would be ultimately responsible for the activities of the managed care organization, but participating physicians would have formal mechanisms for input and responsibilities on crucial medical practice issues.

In addition to the physician's role in making rationing decisions, there is an equally critical role for patients. The decision-making process should include some mechanism for taking into account the preferences and values of the people whom the rationing decisions will most directly affect.[14] Accurate and full disclosure is most important. In addition, a managed care organization could use "town meetings" and other mechanisms whereby subscribers could voice their preferences or "vote" on what treatments should be included in their benefits package.

Once guidelines and criteria are developed at the policy level, physicians are free to make clinical decisions based on those guidelines and criteria. For example, if a managed care plan decided to offer LOCM only to patients at high risk for an adverse reaction to HOCM, physicians would decide which patients are at high risk.

In addition to the development of appropriate procedures for making allocation decisions, there are other steps that must be taken to protect patient welfare when the allocation procedures are implemented. For example, as part of the process of giving patients informed consent to treatment, physicians should disclose all available treatment alternatives, regardless of cost, including those potentially beneficial treatments that are not offered under the terms of the plan. As described in the Council's report on financial incentives to limit care,[1] obligations of disclosure always apply to the physician practicing in managed care. With full understanding of the limitations affecting their treatment, patients will have the opportunity to make alternative arrangements for care that is not available in their health plan. Thus, for example, if the health plan did not cover a particular pharmaceutical that the physician might otherwise have prescribed, the patient could choose to pay out-of-pocket for the pharmaceutical.

It is also critical for managed care plans to have a well-structured appeals process through which physicians and patients can challenge the denial of a particular diagnostic test or therapeutic procedure. Such a process should afford the physician an opportunity to advocate on the patient's behalf before the plan's medical board or governing board. Appeals mechanisms for treatment denials are essential because policy-level allocation decisions can never fully account for all contingencies and will sometimes underserve individual patients. Managed care plans, as institutions, have an ethical responsibility to allow patients to challenge treatment decisions that directly affect their health and well-being.

In some circumstances physicians have an obligation to initiate appeals on behalf of their patients. Cases may arise in which a health plan has an allocation guideline that is generally fair but in particular circumstances results in unfair denials of care, ie, denial of care that would materially benefit the patient. In such cases, the physician's duty as patient advocate requires that the physician challenge the denial and argue for the provision of treatment in the specific case. Cases may also arise in which a health plan has an allocation guideline that is generally unfair in its operation. In such cases, the physician's duty as patient advocate requires not only a challenge to any denials of treatment from the guideline but also advocacy at the health plan's policymaking level to seek an elimination or modification of the guideline.

Conflicts Between Physician and Patient

Ethical Problems With Financial Incentives to Limit Care. As discussed herein, managed care plans encourage physicians to be more cost conscious by using bonuses, fee withholds, and other financial incentives to limit care. With these incentives, physicians recognize that they may reduce their income when they order tests, hospitalize patients, or provide other services. The incentives are not inherently unethical, but they can be depending on their design and intensity.

There are two important ways in which financial incentives to limit care compromise the physician's duty of loyalty to patient care. First, physicians have an incentive to cut corners in their patient care, by temporizing too long, eschewing extra diagnostic tests, or refraining from an expensive referral. Several studies have tried to measure the health outcomes of patients in managed care or prepaid settings against the health outcomes of patients in fee-for-service arrangements. Although disturbing anecdotes abound, these studies have found largely mixed results[16]: harm or inadequate health outcomes have not been conclusively demonstrated in managed care arrangements,[17,18] although these patients may be at an increased risk of harm.[19-21] Second, even in the absence of actual patient harm, the incentives may erode patient trust as patients wonder whether they are receiving all necessary care or are being denied care because of the physicians' pecuniary concerns.

Physicians must place patients' interests ahead of their own interests, including financial remuneration.[1] Financial conflicts are inherent in the practice of medicine, regardless of the system of delivery, and physicians generally have been able to maintain their duty to patient welfare despite those conflicts. However, incentives to limit care are more problematic than incentives to provide care.

First, financial incentives to limit care exploit the financial motive of physicians, making the physician's financial self-interest indispensable for the success of the managed care organization. Second, financial incentives to limit care are less likely than financial incentives created by fee-for-service to coincide with patients' interests, because patients generally prefer the risk of too much care to the risk of too little care. Third, the effects of incentives to limit care are less likely to be noticed by patients. When a physician recommends a course of action under fee-for-service reimbursement, the patient can seek a second opinion. However, when a physician does not offer an intervention under managed care, the patient may have no idea that a treatment option was withheld and therefore not recognize the need for a second opinion.[8]

Not all financial incentives to limit care create the same conflict of interest between the physician's and patient's interests. In general, the greater the strength of the incentive, the more likely it will create a serious conflict of interest that could lead to patient harm. The strength of a financial incentive to limit care can be judged by various factors, including the percentage of the physician's income placed at risk, the frequency with which incentive payments are calculated, and the size of the group of physicians on which the economic performance is judged.[22]

If the managed care plan places 20% of a physician's income at risk, the physician likely will be much more conscious of costs than if the plan places 5% of income at risk. Similarly, if a physician's incentive payments are based solely on his or her treatment decisions, there is a strong incentive to limit services for each patient. When payments are based on the performance of a group of physicians, on the other hand, the incentive is diminished. When physicians are placed at risk together, they have an incentive to ensure that their colleagues are practicing in a cost-effective manner and the incentive payments will be based on costs incurred by a large patient pool. When the patient panel is small, there is a risk that treatment costs will be skewed by an unrepresentative group of patients that have unusually high-cost needs for medical care.

The strength of a financial incentive can also vary with the frequency of incentive payments. If payments are made on a monthly basis rather than a yearly basis, the physician receives rapid feedback on the economic consequences of treatment decisions and is therefore likely to be more sensitive to those consequences. In addition, when incentives are calculated on a monthly basis, there is less of an opportunity for the costs of cases that are above average to be offset by the costs of cases that are below average. Accordingly there is a stronger incentive not to incur unusually high expenses in any one case. Because of this concern, the Health Care Financing Administration, in its rules, would permit managed care plans to place less of their physicians' income at risk if the plans calculate their incentive payments more frequently than once a year.[23]

Preserving the Physician's Role. Before the Council discusses its recommendations for dealing with financial incentives to limit care, it is important to mention that the AMA is precluded from issuing restrictive guidelines in this area. A Federal Trade Commission order that was upheld by the US Supreme Court prohibits the AMA from "regulating" or "advising on the ethical propriety of… the consideration offered or provided to any physician in any contract with any entity that offers physicians' services to the public."[24]

The most effective way to eliminate inappropriate conflicts is to create the use of financial incentives based on quality rather than quantity of services. Reimbursement that serves to promote a standard of "appropriate" behavior helps to maintain the goals of professionalism. Unlike incentives based on quantity of services, which punish the provision of both appropriate and inappropriate services, incentives based on quality of care punish only inappropriate services.

Judgments about the quality of a physician's practice should reflect several measures. First, it is essential to consider objective outcomes data, including data about mortality and morbidity, corrected for caseload. Second, because outcomes are often beyond the physician's control, it is important to consider the degree to which the physician adheres to practice guidelines or other standards of care. Third, patient satisfaction should be considered. Although patients are limited in their ability to evaluate physician competence, they are the best judges of one critical quality of physician care, the physician's bedside manner. In addition, patient satisfaction reflects the extent to which the physician has accommodated the goals of the patient, as required by the patient's right to exercise self-determination in medical care. Fourth, the judgments of a physician's peers should be considered; these judgments provide an important assessment of quality that may be particularly useful "in areas that are difficult to assess reliably with other measures."[25 (p1658)]

Because measurements of quality are still in the rudimentary stages of development, it is important to ensure that other safeguards are in place to prevent abuse from incentives based on quantity of care. Reasonable limits should be placed on the extent to which a physician's ordering of services can affect his or her income. For example, quantitative financial incentives should be calculated on groups of physicians rather than individual physicians.

Patient Autonomy and Responsibility

Many commentators argue that managed care threatens patient autonomy because it curtails patients' freedom of choice. Patients are usually limited in their choice of primary care physicians and, to a much greater degree, specialists, and they are sometimes limited in their choice of treatments. Patients may not be able to receive a desired diagnostic test or referral, and their freedom to personally tailor treatment can be thwarted.
In addition, continuity of care may be disrupted if a patient is forced, for a variety of reasons, to change physicians to keep their health care benefits.[26]

Public participation in the formulation of benefits packages may resolve some of these concerns about limited autonomy. Legislation reasonably protecting patients' rights to be informed and to choose and protecting physicians' rights to remain professionals is also essential. Patients can exercise their autonomy by participating in the decisions of their health plan or in government processes that may restrict their choices or benefits. In addition, patients have a responsibility to learn as much as they can about their choices of plans, including the exact nature of the different benefits packages and their limitations. Patients have a responsibility to make sure they know and understand the terms of their own health care plan.

As patient advocates, physicians continue to have duties of disclosure. They must ensure that all treatment alternatives, regardless of cost, are disclosed. They must also ensure that the managed care organization has fulfilled its obligation to disclose the terms of the benefits package, including all limitations and restrictions.

Patient autonomy does not guarantee the right to have all treatment choices funded. Some limits on personal freedom are inevitable in a society that tries to provide all of its members with adequate health care. The desire for accurate diagnosis and use of technological medical care, no matter how little the benefit, has been cited as a major factor in increasing health care costs in this country.[27] Moreover, patient autonomy entails patient responsibility, including a responsibility to abide by societal decisions to conserve health care and to make an individual effort to use resources wisely and lead a healthy lifestyle.

While physicians must remain patient advocates, patients do not have an unlimited claim to physicians' obligation to provide health care. Physicians should not manipulate or "game" the system to answer patients" demands.[28]

To fully exercise their autonomy, patients need to be fully informed about the philosophy and goals of managed care. In an earlier report, the Council stated that the physician's responsibilities under managed care include a duty to disclose to the patient conflicts of interest that may affect patient care and medical alternatives that cannot be offered because of the restrictions of the managed care plan. That report specifically states that physicians have a duty to disclose financial incentives, to disclose contractual agreements restricting referral, and to ensure that the managed care plan makes adequate disclosure of the details of the plan to subscribers.[1,29]

Guidelines

For the reasons described in this report, the Council on Ethical and Judicial Affairs issues the following guidelines:

1. The duty of patient advocacy is a fundamental element of the patient-physician relationship that should not be altered by the system of health care delivery in which physicians practice. Physicians must continue to place the interests of their patients first.

2. When managed care plans place restrictions on the care that physicians in the plan may provide to their patients, the following principles should be followed:

   (a) Any broad allocation guidelines that restrict care and choices which go beyond the cost-benefit judgments made by physicians as a part of their normal professional responsibilities should be established at a policymaking level so that individual physicians are not asked to engage in ad hoc bedside rationing.

   (b) Regardless of any allocation guidelines or gatekeeper directives, physicians must advocate for any care they believe will materially benefit their patients.

(c) Physicians should be given an active role in contributing their expertise to any allocation process and should advocate for guidelines that are sensitive to differences among patients. Managed care plans should create structures similar to hospital medical staffs that allow physicians to have meaningful input into the plan's development of allocation guidelines. Guidelines for allocating health care should be reviewed on a regular basis and updated to reflect advances in medical knowledge and changes in relative costs.

(d) Adequate appellate mechanisms for both patients and physicians should be in place to address disputes regarding medically necessary care. In some circumstances, physicians have an obligation to initiate appeals on behalf of their patients. Cases may arise in which a health plan has an allocation guideline that is generally fair but in particular circumstances results in unfair denials of care, ie, denial of care that, in the physician's judgment, would materially benefit the patient. In such cases, the physician's duty as patient advocate requires that the physician challenge the denial and argue for the provision of treatment in the specific case. Cases may also arise in which a health plan has an allocation guideline that is generally unfair in its operation. In such cases, the physician's duty as patient advocate requires not only a challenge to any denials of treatment from the guideline but also advocacy at the health plan's policymaking level to seek an elimination or modification of the guideline. Physicians should assist patients who wish to seek additional appropriate care outside the plan when the physician believes the care is in the patient's best interests.

(e) Managed care plans must adhere to the requirement of informed consent that patients be given full disclosure of material information. Full disclosure requires that managed care plans inform potential subscribers of limitations or restrictions on the benefits package when they are considering entering the plan.

(f) Physicians also should continue to promote full disclosure to patients enrolled in managed care organizations. The physician's obligation to disclose treatment alternatives to patients is not altered by any limitations in the coverage provided by the patient's managed care plan. Full disclosure includes informing patients of all their treatment options, even those that may not be covered under the terms of the managed care plan. Patients may then determine whether an appeal is appropriate or whether they wish to seek care outside the plan for treatment alternatives that are not covered.

(g) Physicians should not participate in any plan that encourages or requires care at or below minimum professional standards.

3. When physicians are employed or reimbursed by managed care plans that offer financial incentives to limit care, serious potential conflicts are created between the physicians' personal financial interests and the needs of their patients. Efforts to contain health care costs should not place patient welfare at risk. Thus, financial incentives are permissible only if they promote the cost-effective delivery of health care and not the withholding of medically necessary care.

(a) Any incentives to limit care must be disclosed fully to patients by plan administrators on enrollment and at least annually thereafter.

(b) Limits should be placed on the magnitude of fee withholds, bonuses, and other financial incentives to limit care. Calculating incentive payments according to the performance of a sizable group of physicians rather than on an individual basis should be encouraged.

(c) Health plans or other groups should develop financial incentives based on quality of care. Such incentives should complement financial incentives based on the quantity of services used.

4. Patients have an individual responsibility to be aware of the benefits and limitations of their health care coverage. Patients should exercise their autonomy by public participation in the formulation of benefits packages and by prudent selection of health care coverage that best suits their needs.

Report of the Council on Ethical and Judicial Affairs of the American Medical Association.
June 1994.

Endnotes

1. Council on Ethical and Judicial Affairs, American Medical Association. Financial incentives to limit care: financial implications for HMOs and IPAs. In: *Code of Medical Ethics: Reports of the Ethical and Judicial Affairs of the American Medical Association, Vol I.* Chicago: American Medical Association; 1990:130-135. See also, Council on Ethical and Judicial Affairs, American Medical Association. The ethical implications of capitation. In: *Proceedings of the House of Delegates of the American Medical Association:* 146th Annual Meeting. Chicago: American Medical Association; 1997:268-273 and, Council on Ethical and Judicial Affairs, American Medical Association. Financial incentives and the practice of medicine. In: *Proceedings of the House of Delegates of the American Medical Association:* 51st Interim Meeting. Chicago: American Medical Association; 1997.

2. Enthoven A, Kronick R. A consumer-choice health plan for the 1990s: universal health insurance in a system designed to promote quality and economy. *N Engl J Med.* 1989;320:29-37.

3. Povar C, Moreno J. Hippocrates and the health maintenance organization. *Ann Intern Med.* 1988 109:419-424.

4. Iglehart JK. The American health care system: managed care. *N Engl J Med.* 1992;327:742-747.

5. American Medical Association. *Principles of Managed Care: A Summary of American Medical Association Policy.* Chicago: American Medical Association, 1993.

6. Council on Ethical and Judicial Affairs, American Medical Association. Ethical issues involved in the growing AIDS crisis. *JAMA.* 1988;259:1360-1361.

7. Relman AS. Medical practice under the Clinton reforms. *N Engl J Med.* 1993;329:1574-1576.

8. Morreim EH. Cost containment: challenging fidelity and justice. *Hastings Cent Rep.* 1988;18(6):20-25.

9. American Medical Association. How cost containment may affect the standard of care in medical malpractice litigation. In: *Proceedings of the House of Delegates of the American Medical Association: 40th Annual Meeting.* Chicago: American Medical Association; 1991:121-136.

10. Bettman MA. Ionic versus nonionic contrast agents for intravenous use: are all the answers in? *Radiology.* 1990;175:616-618.

11. Katayama H, Yamaguchi K, Kozuka T, Takashima T, Seez P, Matsuura K. Adverse reactions to ionic and nonionic contrast media: a report from the Japanese Committee on the Safety of Contrast Media. *Radiology.* 1990;175:621-628.

12. Peters WP, Rogers MC. Variation in approval by insurance companies of coverage for autologous bone marrow transplantation for breast cancer. *N Engl J Med.* 1994;330:473-477.

13. Pellegrino ED. Rationing health care: the ethics of medical gatekeeping. *J Contemp Health Law Policy.* 1986;2:23-45.

14. Council on Ethical and Judicial Affairs, American Medical Association. Ethical issues in health care system reform: the provision of adequate health care. *JAMA.* 1994;272:1056-1062.

15. American Medical Association. *Physician Health Plans and Networks Act of 1994.* Chicago: American Medical Association; 1994.

16. Miller RH, Luft HS. Managed care plan performance since 1980: a literature analysis. *JAMA.* 1994,271:1512-1519.

17. Rubenstein LV, Kahn KL, Reinisch E, et al. Changes in quality of care for five diseases measured by implicit review, 1981 to 1981. *JAMA.* 1990; 264:1974-1979.

18. Kahn KL, Keeler EB, Sherwood ML, et al. Comparing outcomes of care before and after implementation of the DRG-based prospective payment system. *JAMA.* 1990;261:1984-1988.

19. Kosecoff J, Kahn KL, Rogers WH, et al. Prospective payment system and impairment at discharge: the "quicker-and-sicker" story revisited. *JAMA.* 1990;264:1980-1983.

20. Ware JE Jr, Brook RH, Rogers WH, et al. Comparison of health outcomes at a health maintenance organization with those of fee-for-service. *Lancet.* 1986;1:1017-1022.

21. Clement DG, Retchin SM, Brown RS, Stegall MH. Access and outcomes of elderly patients enrolled in managed care. *JAMA.* 1994;271:1487-1192.

22. US General Accounting Office. *Medicare: Physician Incentive Payments by Prepaid Health Plans Could Lower Quality of Care.* Washington, DC: US Government Printing Office; 1988:23-27.

23. Health Care Financing Administration, US Dept of Health and Human Services. *Medicare and Medicaid programs: requirements for physician incentive plans in prepaid health care organizations.* Federal Register. 1992;57:59024-59040.

24. Federal Trade Commission Order. Docket No. 9064. *JAMA.* 1982;248:981-982.

25. Ramsey PG, Wenrich MD, Carline JD, Inui TS, Larson EB, LoGerfo JP. Use of peer ratings to evaluate physician performance. *JAMA.* 1993;269:1660-1665.

26. Emanuel EJ, Brett AS. Managed competition and the patient-physician relationship. *N Engl J Med.* 1993;329:879-882.

27. Kassirer JP. Our stubborn quest for diagnostic certainty: a cause of excessive testing. *N Engl J Med.* 1989;320:1489-1491.

28. Morreim EH. Gaming the system: dodging the rules, ruling the dodgers. *Arch Intern Med.* 1991;151:443-447.

29. Council on Ethical and Judicial Affairs, American Medical Association. Opinion 8.13: referral of patients' disclosure of limitations. In: *Code of Medical Ethics: Current Opinion With Annotations.* Chicago: American Medical Association; 1994.

Managed Care Cost Containment Involving Prescription Drugs

In an earlier report, the Council on Ethical and Judicial Affairs discussed the ethical tensions placed on physicians by the cost containment techniques of managed care.[1] As managed care plans strive to meet the needs of society to restrain the growth of health care costs and to allocate health care fairly among different patients, the physician's duty of loyalty to patients may be unduly compromised. Excessive pressure may be imposed on physicians to preserve resources for other patients and to withhold too much care from individual patients they are treating. Financial incentives to limit care may pressure physicians to sacrifice patient welfare to protect their own financial security. The Council concluded that allocation decisions should be made at a policy-making level, at which physicians provide their expertise, so that allocation decisions need not be made at the bedside. The Council also recommended that limitations be placed on the kinds of financial incentives that are used by managed care plans.

In this report, the Council addresses efforts to limit the cost of prescription drugs. It is important that these efforts be designed in ways that do not compromise patient welfare or the integrity of the patient-physician relationship.

Formularies—limited lists of approved pharmaceuticals—are the most prevalent means of containing drug costs and are utilized by most managed care plans. In a formulary system, if a physician prescribes a drug that is not on the formulary list, the plan ordinarily will not cover the cost of the drug. The needs of specific patients may be ignored in this framework, because approved drugs are selected on the basis of average patient outcome, not individual effectiveness. Patients may not be duly informed of formulary implications, either in advance of enrolling in the plan or on a prescription-to-prescription basis. There is also the potential for doctors to sacrifice optimal therapeutic treatment for the benefits of cost-containment.

Other managed care strategies threaten patient welfare as well. Prior authorization procedures can be cumbersome for physicians, prescription caps can be unduly restrictive for patients with chronic conditions, and excessive copayments can block access to optimal treatment. As large pharmaceutical manufacturers purchase pharmaceutical benefit management companies (PBMs), the manufacturers may use their control to ensure that their products are given priority when decisions are made about including or excluding drugs from the formularies. In addition, personal financial incentives have been used to encourage physicians to switch patients to different drugs, pitting the interests of patients against the economic interests of their health care providers.

Managed care plans also have used techniques to encourage switches to a different drug without ensuring adequate disclosure of the benefits and risks of the different drug to the patient.

Pharmaceutical Industry Relationships

As managed care plans increasingly limit prescription drug costs through formularies, volume discounts, and other techniques, pharmaceutical manufacturers have countered with measures to preserve or enhance their bargaining power.[2] Since managed care plans often use generic versions of pharmaceuticals to keep costs down, manufacturers of brand-name drugs have expanded their activities into the production of generic drugs. There also have been some efforts by drug companies to exercise greater control over prescribing by managing health maintenance organizations (HMOs).[3] Perhaps the most troublesome trend has been the purchase of drug benefit management companies by pharmaceutical companies.[4]

Pharmaceutical benefit management companies contract with managed care organizations, insurance companies and employer health plans to oversee prescription plans. They offer cost-effective management of formularies and accumulate data on prescribing practices, price controls, and therapeutic effectiveness to determine where cost savings can be realized. Pharmaceutical benefit managers coordinate drug coverage for 44% of the American population.[5] This figure is expected to grow.

PBMs became the focus of public attention in 1993 when Merck bought one of the leading PBMs, Medco Containment Services. Other multi-billion dollar agreements followed, including SmithKline Beecham's acquisition of Diversified Pharmaceutical Services and Eli Lilly's purchase of PCS Health Systems. These three pharmaceutical benefit managers oversee prescriptions for more than 100 million Americans.[6i] There appeared to be a clear conflict of interest in such consolidation, presumably because drug companies would want the PBMs they purchase to give preference to their products in promotion and marketing. The Federal Trade Commission (FTC), concerned about possible antitrust violations, undertook review of these transactions. The Food and Drug Administration (FDA) also expressed concern over the influence of pharmaceutical manufacturers on the managed care drug distributors they had acquired. The FDA contacted Eli Lilly, Merck, and SmithKline Beecham, admonishing them to neither pressure doctors to prescribe drugs that are not medically indicated nor withhold sufficient disclosures to patients regarding the risks of adverse side effects.[7]

Fears that formularies would be compromised may be exaggerated; in a competitive market, a PBM could not make concessions for the parent company unless the concessions were in fact the most cost-effective measures available. Nevertheless, PBMs' access to valuable industry data would be advantageous for any pharmaceutical company, particularly when trying to prove its drugs more cost-effective than those of their competitors.[8]

FTC monitors closely scrutinized the Eli Lilly deal and finally gave conditional approval.[9] Under the agreement, the FTC required that PCS Health Systems remain open to competitors' products and that Lilly build a "fire wall" to keep it from obtaining other companies' pricing information, particularly when bids for formulary inclusion are being considered. These requirements may prevent undue influence by drug manufacturers in the formulary decisions of their subsidiary PBMs and may also discourage other manufacturers from purchasing PBMs. It remains unclear, however, how the FTC intends to monitor and enforce compliance with these provisions.

The FTC is reconsidering prior deals and may impose similar requirements on the companies involved. Of particular interest is Merck, which announced a 15% increase in fourth-quarter earnings,[10] crediting a rise in Merck drugs on Medco formularies. Merck's share of Medco's recommended drugs rose from less than 10% to 12%.[11]

In sum, consolidation in the pharmaceutical industry may provide an unfair competitive advantage to pharmaceutical manufacturers that own PBMs. FTC requirements may provide a sufficient safeguard against abuse. If not, then it may be necessary to prohibit manufacturers from purchasing PBMs entirely.

Use of Formularies and Other Cost Containment Mechanisms

The Typical Design of Formularies. The evolution of formularies has had an impact on care in a variety of clinical settings, and it largely preceded the boom of managed care. Formulary systems were first adopted in hospitals to limit the variety of drugs a hospital pharmacy needed to keep in stock. Since the 1993 Omnibus Budget Reconciliation Act,[12] formularies have also been applied to state Medicaid programs.[13] Most recently, they were proposed as part of the Clinton health plan's Medicare prescription drug benefit.[14] They have had the greatest effect, however, on HMOs, preferred provider organizations (PPOs), and other managed care constructs.

Formularies derive from formulary systems, a method whereby the medical staff of an institution evaluates, appraises and selects drugs considered to be most useful in patient care.[15] In most managed care formulary systems, a pharmacy and therapeutics (P&T) committee is appointed to review candidates for the formulary, generally considering a variety of drugs from the same class and selecting the most cost-effective for inclusion. Physicians participating in the plan are bound to prescribe drugs from that formulary. If patients choose to go outside a formulary, they may be subject to a higher copayment or may even be held responsible for the full cost of the prescribed drug. Physicians can request additions to formularies, and accommodations can be made in exceptional cases for provision of non-formulary drugs. While the percentage of HMOs that allow for physician overrides of formularies is increasing,[16] there is little or no data on the percentage of requests for additions or exceptions that actually are approved. Managed care plans benefit from adherence in formulary systems because they can ensure that their patient care funds are not spent on unnecessarily expensive drugs. In addition, by ordering fewer drugs at a higher volume per drug, they can negotiate more favorable terms with the pharmaceutical companies. Indeed, discounts can be as much as 10% of a drug's cost.[17] Plans encourage physicians and plan-affiliated pharmacists to adhere to formularies by linking their compensation or status in the plan to their prescribing practices, or simply by making it more costly for patients if physicians deviate from the formulary.

Physicians, pharmacists, plan executives, and benefit managers are the most regular participants on P&T committees, that determine formularies. Ideally, committee representatives are independent from plan influence and are elected by the plan's medical executive committee, much like the medical staff organization. In some cases, the position may be too time-consuming for volunteers. When it is necessary to hire committee members, the administrative structure may be bypassed and recommendations may go directly to the Board. The P&T committee usually assesses drugs to determine therapeutic equivalence. Once satisfied that the considered drugs do not vary significantly in therapeutic benefit, P&T committees often will put the drug slot out for bid, choosing the drug (or drugs) for which the best terms are offered by the pharmaceutical company. In making their choice, P&T committees consider presentations from drug company representatives, who offer clinical trials and outcome analyses to demonstrate cost-effectiveness.

There are a variety of established mechanisms for reducing the costs of prescription drugs. The first is therapeutic interchange, where a related, but less expensive drug will be substituted for its costly counterpart. This practice recognizes the proliferation of so-called "me-too" drugs that replicate the action of already established drugs. Another is generic substitution, where the brand-name drug will be replaced by its generic form. According to recent published data, some 40% of all HMO prescriptions are generics, compared with 20% outside HMOs.[18] Current use of generic drugs is likely higher. Also, 64% of HMO plans use therapeutic equivalent strategies and 96% use generic substitution to varying degrees.[16]

To monitor these efforts, virtually all institutions create review mechanisms to ensure that the formulary is up to date and is affording appropriate patient care. Reviews are generally conducted on at least a quarterly basis.[15] The drug use evaluation (DUE) or drug utilization review (DUR) committees play instrumental roles in the proper application of formulary policy. These entities oversee establishment and use of drug therapy management protocols, organize periodic review of drug use statistics by the P&T committee, monitor pharmacist intervention, and evaluate drug-dispensing habits of individual medical staffs.[19] In addition, there should be a mechanism for ongoing peer review of formulary policy.

The vast majority of HMOs utilize formularies to contain drug costs.[15,20] There, however, are a variety of formulary system configurations being employed in the managed care industry. Some HMOs still adhere to "open" formularies, where less expensive and therapeutically similar drugs are recommended to participating providers, but the option to prescribe outside the formulary still exists. Usually these plans offer coverage for drugs off the formulary, possibly charging a higher copayment. The current trend is towards "closed" formularies, where only the drugs on the list can be prescribed unless patients are willing to pay for a nonformulary drug themselves. Other cost-containment efforts include maximum allowable costs (MACs), which specify upper limits for payment of prescription ingredient costs, and prior authorization, where coverage depends on prior approval for prescribing or dispensing.

Previous AMA policy has addressed the practicalities of formulary structures.[21] These policies have advocated the establishment of formularies in inpatient hospital and selected outpatient settings where there is an established P&T committee and concurrence of organized medical staff. Therapeutic interchange, the authorized exchange of therapeutic alternates in accordance with previously approved guidelines, also was recognized. Finally, AMA policy requires provision of protocols for timely procurement of nonformulary drug products prescribed by a physician for the individualized care of a specific patient. The AMA's policies are intended to encourage physicians to supplement medical considerations with cost considerations when selecting the drug of choice for an individual patient and to become well-informed about the quality of prescription drug products available from multiple sources.

Ethical Concerns With Cost Containment Mechanisms. Proponents have argued that streamlining of prescription options has succeeded in containing the growing cost of pharmaceuticals and has resulted in the most appropriate utilization of available drug therapy. But the basic question of whether formularies are truly cost-effective is much debated in managed care analyses.[22] Some commentators believe that prescription of generics or marginally less therapeutic drugs in managed care organizations compromises patient care to the point where any savings are offset by increases in costly office consultations and hospitalizations. The empirical data are inconclusive; while some studies support assertions of cost-effective patient care, other investigations of uncertain validity raise cause for concern.[23] One study of hospital formularies found that limiting a physician's choice of drugs for ulcers, asthma, and hearth conditions saved a marginal amount of money, but hospitalization utilization rose, offsetting any savings. Prior authorization, which requires physicians to secure permission from a specialist or other designated person before using high-cost drugs, can unduly discourage optimal drug therapy. Prior authorization requirements also may increase administrative costs. Managed care organizations sometimes restrain drug costs by imposing prescription caps with provisions for waivers of the caps when justified by a patient's particular circumstances. With a prescription cap, patients ordinarily are limited to a certain number of prescriptions in any month, or other fixed time period, unless their physician receives permission to exceed the cap. Studies have shown that prescription caps without waivers threaten patient welfare. Patients on maintenance drug therapy for chronic conditions are especially endangered when access to pharmaceuticals is limited by a prescription cap. In one study of schizophrenic patients on Medicaid, hospitalizations rose significantly with the introduction of prescription caps.[25]

Formularies, specifically, may compromise patient care in several ways. Necessary pharmaceuticals may be omitted in the process of formulary compilation, either because consolidation results in pharmaceutical manufacturers favoring their own drugs over the drugs of competitors, or because formulary decisions may fail to account sufficiently for variations among individual patients. Some drugs may not provide more benefit than their counterparts on average, but may make a substantial difference to a minority of patients.[26] Eliminating the option of what may be better for some inevitably compromises the care of a small population of patients. In addition, these compromises may not even be offset by cost savings; expenses for a patient who was inadequately treated initially may far outweigh the savings on the drugs with which the patient was treated.

Preventing Ethical Abuses. Physicians should be informed of formulary constraints while negotiating provider contracts. Physicians who participate in managed care plans should maintain awareness of plan decisions about drug selection by staying informed about P&T committee actions and by ongoing personal review of formulary composition. In addition, physicians should recognize that there are risks to patient care from pharmaceutical industry consolidation involving the managed care plans or pharmacy benefit plans with which they deal. Any perceived inappropriate influence on formulary development should be reported to regulatory authorities.

Physicians should be particularly vigilant to ensure that formulary decisions adequately reflect the needs of individual patients and that individual needs are not unfairly sacrificed by decisions based on the needs of the average patient. Physicians are ethically required to advocate for additions to the formulary when they think patients would benefit and for exceptions to the formulary on a case-by-case basis when justified by the health care needs of particular patients. Efficient mechanisms to appeal formulary exclusions should be established.

Other cost-containment mechanisms, including prescription caps and prior authorization, should be designed in ways that do not unduly burden physicians or patients in accessing optimal drug therapy. For example, prescription caps should be liberal and there should be flexible waiver provisions to allow for appropriate exceptions to the caps, so that the threat to patient welfare can be neutralized.

Pressures or Incentives to Limit Prescription Drug Costs

In addition to excluding certain drugs from the plan's formulary, managed care plans control prescription drug costs by encouraging or pressuring physicians to prescribe lower-cost drugs within the formulary or to not prescribe a drug at all. Many of these efforts are an important part of the plan's efforts to contain their health care costs. Physicians who developed their prescribing practices in a fee-for-service environment may not have had sufficient incentive to consider costs when prescribing drugs. Consequently, managed care plans may need to ensure that physicians incorporate cost considerations in their decisions about drug prescribing.

However, some techniques may create undue incentives or pressures. In some cases, physicians are given financial incentives by their managed care plan or the plan's pharmaceutical benefit manager to keep prescribing costs down. For example, end-of-year bonuses may be increased if the physicians minimized the prescription drug costs of their patients, or if they have complied with requests by the plan to switch their patients to lower-cost drugs. Managed care plans also may have plan administrators or pharmacists call physicians about changing prescriptions, and sometimes the frequency and intensity of the calls can reach the level of harassment. Both incentives and pressures are particularly troublesome if the plan sends the message to physicians that failure to comply with requests for prescription changes will jeopardize the physician's participation in the plan. Physicians should guard against acquiescing to switch requests too readily. In some plans, the pharmacist or the plan secures a switch from the doctor and directly notifies the patients that they are to pick up the new drugs at the pharmacy as soon as possible. This approach eliminates the possibility of an informed consent dialogue between the physician and the patient; patients lose the opportunity to receive an explanation or instructions from their physician or to express their preference for the original drug. Of particular concern are plans in which switches are automatic and neither the physician nor the patient is made aware of the change.

While it is not always possible to discern the line between appropriate persuasion and inappropriate harassment, limits need to be placed on the extent to which managed care plans use incentives or pressures to lower prescription drug costs. Financial incentives are permissible when they promote cost-effectiveness, not when they require withholding medically necessary care. Physicians must not be made to feel that they jeopardize their compensation or participation if they prescribe drugs that are necessary for their patients but that also may be costly. In accordance with the Council's report, *Ethical Issues in Managed Care*[1], there should be limits on the magnitude of financial incentives; incentives should be calculated according to the practices of a sizeable group of physicians rather than on an individual basis; and incentives should be based on quality of care rather than cost of care should be used. Prescriptions should not be changed without physicians having a chance to discuss the change with the patient. All fiscal incentives should be disclosed fully to the patient. The American Pharmaceutical Association (APhA) also has supported pharmacist disclosure of incentives to physicians and patients when they propose a switch. This is in keeping with APhA's *Code of Ethics*, which states, "A pharmacist should strive to provide information to patients regarding professional services truthfully, accurately, and fully and should avoid misleading patients regarding the nature, cost or value of these professional services."[27]

Educational efforts can be an important adjunct to financial incentives. Publication of price lists, at the very least, goes a long way to boosting physicians' awareness of cost. Many plans encourage cost-effective prescribing practices by informing physicians of the existence of drugs that provide comparable benefits at lower cost than drugs currently being used. Pharmaceutical benefit managers offer computer technology to access medical information networks that detail the cost and effectiveness of formulary options. In addition, almost two-thirds of HMOs reported automated systems for tracking drug interactions.[16]

Disclosure to Patients

Patients should fully understand the methods used by their managed care plans to limit prescription drug costs. In the course of enrollment, the plan must disclose the existence of formularies, the provisions for cases in which the physician prescribes a drug that is not included in the formulary, and the incentives or other mechanisms used to encourage physicians to consider costs when prescribing drugs. Plans also should disclose any relationships with PBMs or pharmaceutical companies that could influence the composition of the formulary. This information should be included in HMO literature and patient orientations. Any inquiries patients have about inclusion of particular drugs on formularies should be answered prior to enrollment. When physicians do not prescribe a drug that would offer significant advantage to the patient because it is not on the formulary, and they are unable to secure a formulary exception, the physician must disclose that information to the patient.

While some would consider it cruel to disclose treatment options that a patient clearly cannot afford, physicians should never presume that they are acting in their patient's best interest by prescribing the less expensive, less effective drug. It is possible that a patient would be willing to sacrifice some other expense to pay out-of-pocket for a drug that may give a better, sustained quality of life. As Morreim notes, "the patient's right to self-determination encompasses the right to decide one's budget as well as one's body."[28] A doctor should not assume that the patient cannot afford an opportunity for better outcome. As with any managed care restriction, if patients do not like a particular recommended course of treatment, they have the option to disenroll from the plan or pay out-of-pocket for an alternative. Physicians must become more comfortable weighing these cost-benefit issues with their patients.

Involving patients in specific prescription decisions can be very helpful. Studies have shown that, when patients have been thoroughly educated about the expenses involved and the therapeutic comparability of two drugs, they are generally receptive to accepting the more cost-effective drug.[29] Such preliminary studies should encourage physicians to include their patients in prescribing choices.

Conclusion

In the case of prescription drugs, the AMA in the past has encouraged physicians to supplement medical judgment with cost considerations in drug selection. Managed care organizations establish drug formulary systems for this purpose. To ensure optimal patient care, various ethical requirements must be established for formulary application. The AMA's Council on Ethical and Judicial Affairs offers the following recommendations:

- Physicians who participate in managed care plans should maintain awareness of plan decisions about drug selection by staying informed about pharmacy and therapeutics (P&T) committee actions and by ongoing personal review of formulary composition. P&T committee members should include independent physician representatives. Mechanisms should be established for ongoing peer review of formulary policy. Physicians who perceive inappropriate influence on formulary development from pharmaceutical industry consolidation should notify the proper regulatory authorities.

- Physicians should be particularly vigilant to ensure that formulary decisions adequately reflect the needs of individual patients and that individual needs are not unfairly sacrificed by decisions based on the needs of the average patient. Physicians are ethically required to advocate for additions to the formulary when they think patients would benefit materially and for exceptions to the formulary on a case-by-case basis when justified by the health care needs of particular patients. Mechanisms to appeal formulary exclusions should be established. Other cost-containment mechanisms, including prescription caps and prior authorization, should not unduly burden physicians or patients in accessing optimal drug therapy.

- Limits should be placed on the extent to which managed care plans use incentives or pressures to lower prescription drug costs. Financial incentives are permissible when they promote cost-effectiveness, not when they require withholding medically necessary care. Physicians must not be made to feel that they jeopardize their compensation or participation in a managed care plan if they prescribe drugs that are necessary for their patients but that also may be costly. There should be limits on the magnitude of financial incentives, incentives should be calculated according to the practices of a sizeable group of physicians rather than on an individual basis, and incentives based on quality of care rather than cost of care should be used. Prescriptions should not be changed without physicians having a chance to discuss the change with the patient.

- Managed care plans should develop and implement educational programs on cost-effective prescribing practices. Such initiatives are preferable to financial incentives or pressures by HMOs or hospitals, which can be ethically problematic.

- Patients must fully understand the methods used by their managed care plans to limit prescription drug costs. During enrollment, the plan must disclose the existence of formularies, the provisions for cases in which the physician prescribes a drug that is not included in the formulary and the incentives or other mechanisms used to encourage physicians to consider costs when prescribing drugs. In addition, plans should disclose any relationships with pharmaceutical benefit management companies or pharmaceutical companies that could influence the composition of the formulary. If physicians exhaust all avenues to secure a formulary exception for a significantly advantageous drug, they are still obligated to disclose the option of the more beneficial, more costly drug to the patient, so that the patient can decide whether to pay out-of-pocket.

- Research should be conducted to assess the impact on patient welfare of formulary activity and other approaches to containing prescription drug costs.

Report of the Council on Ethical and Judicial Affairs of the American Medical Association.
June 1995. (*FDLI.* 1998;53:25-34.)

Endnotes

1. Council on Ethical and Judicial Affairs, American Medical Association. Ethical issues in managed care. *JAMA.* 1995;273:330-335

2. McGahan A. Focus on pharmaceuticals; industry structure and competitive advantage. *Harvard Business Review.* November-December 1994;115-124.

3. Borzo G. Searle joins in pushing managed care for elderly. *American Medical News.* February 6, 1995:12.

4. Tanouye E, Steinmetz C. Managed-care feeding frenzy probably hasn't ended. *Wall Street Journal.* July 13, 1994:B3.

5. Freudenheim M. Drug merger chill? *New York Times.* October 27, 1994:D2.

6. Tanouye E, Anders G. Drug industry takeovers mean more cost-cutting, less research spending. *Wall Street Journal.* February 1, 1995:B1.

7. Freudenheim M. FDA cautions 3 drug makers on pressure. *New York Times.* February 1, 1995:D3.

8. Tanouye E. Owning Medco, Merck takes drug marketing the next logical step. *Wall Street Journal.* May 31, 1994:A1.

9. Freudenheim M. Eli Lilly deal is advanced by the FTC. *New York Times.* November 5, 1994:Cl.

10. Winslow R. Merck 4th-quarter earnings rose 15%, helped by Zocor drug, managed care. *Wall Street Journal.* January 25, 1995:B8.

11. Tanouye E. Merck officials say Medco deal aiding growth. *Wall Street Journal.* November 30, 1994:B6.

12. Omnibus Reconciliation Act, Pub L No 103-66,107 Stat 312:1992.

13. Intergovernmental Health Policy Project. *Pharmaceuticals: an overview of 1994 state legislative activity,* 1994 Legislative Tracking Service. George Washington University. 1994.

14. Goldberg R. AARP hands members a poison pill. *Wall Street Journal.* August 16, 1994:A12.

15. Board of Trustees of the American Medical Association. *Drug Formularies and Therapeutic Interchange.* In: *Proceedings of the American Medical Association House of Delegates:* 47th Interim Meeting. Chicago: American Medical Association. 1993:155-148

16. Marion Merrel Dow. *Managed Care Digest.* HMO Edition. 1994.

17. Mandelker J. Controlling the cost of branded drugs; use of formularies. *Business and Health.* 1993;11(13):44.

18. Winslow R. Prescribing decisions increasingly are made by the cost-conscious. *Wall Street Journal.* December 25, 1992:1A.

19. Cotterell C, Dombroske L, Fischermann E. Comprehensive drug-use evaluation program in a health maintenance organization. *Am J of Hosp Pharm.* 1991;48:1712-1717.

20. Gabel J, Dial T, Hobart J, Pan L, Bergsten C, Bernstein A, et al for the Group Health Association of America. *HMO Industry Profile.* Washington, DC; 1994.

21. American Medical Association. Policy 125.000. In: *American Medical Association Policy Compendium.* Chicago: American Medical Association. 1994.

22. HMO pharmacy cost management techniques questioned by NPC outcomes study. FDC Reports. *The Green Sheet.* 1994;43(38):2.

23. Knowlton C, Knapp D. Community pharmacists help HMO cut drug costs. *Am Pharm.* 1994;34:36-42.

24. Sloan FA, et al. Hospital drug formularies and use of hospital services. Medicare. 1993;10:31

25. Soumerai S, McLaughlin T, Ross-Degnan D, Casteris C, Bollini P. Effects of limiting Medicaid drug-reimbursement benefits on the use of psychotropic agents and acute mental health services by patients with schizophrenia. *N Engl J Med.* 1994;331:650-655.

26. Morreim EH. New duties in the medical standard of care. *J of Legal Medicine.* 1991;12:275-329.

27. American Pharmaceutical Association. *Code of Ethics.* (Rev. ed. 1981.)

28. Morreim EH. Fiscal scarcity and the inevitability of bedside budget balancing. *Arch Int Med.* 1989;149:1012-1015.

29. McDonough K, Weaver R, Viall G. Enalapril to lisinopril: Economic impact of a voluntary angio converting enzyme-inhibitor substitution program in a staff-model health maintenance organization. *Annals of Pharmacotherapy.* 1992;26:399-404.

Restrictions on Disclosure in Managed Care Contracts

The changes that have characterized the movement to reform the country's health care system have presented the medical profession with the task of providing guidelines that reaffirm the ethical absolutes of medicine within the context of new and shifting health care delivery structures. One of the most fundamental of these ethical absolutes is the right of patients to complete information concerning their condition and treatment.[1] In a previous report, the Council included this right in its broader discussion of the ethical issues surrounding managed care, writing in part, "Physicians also should continue to promote full disclosure to patients enrolled in managed care organizations."[2] The Council built on that premise, stating, "The physician's obligation to disclose treatment alternatives to patients is not altered by any limitations in the coverage provided by the patient's managed care plan."

Clauses that Restrict Disclosure

Despite the unambiguous ethical requirements demanding full disclosure, some managed care organizations include clauses in their employment contracts which directly inhibit the ability of physicians to keep their patients fully informed. These contract clauses, labeled "gag clauses" by some observers, are qualitatively different from other confidentiality clauses designed to protect proprietary information from competitors. While these latter clauses legitimately safeguard business interests, "gag clauses" erect inappropriate barriers to necessary communications between physicians and patients.

Probably the most problematic restrictive language in contracts is found in general statements which prohibit physicians from making statements to patients which could negatively impact their perception of the health plan. For example, one HMO included in its contract the following language: "Physician shall agree not to take any action or make any communication which undermines or could undermine the confidence of enrollees, potential enrollees, their employers, their unions, or the public in (HMO) or the quality of (HMO) coverage." Clauses containing general prohibitions such as this can easily be interpreted to encompass disclosure of treatment options not covered by the contracting plan as such disclosure could cause patients to seek an alternative plan more suitably tailored to their health needs. Because complete disclosure could have economic consequences for a plan by contributing to patient attrition, there is an incentive to restrict the ability of physicians to provide patients with certain information. However, contract language which so prioritizes the financial success of a plan over the right of patients to all relevant medical information cannot be reconciled with the fundamental ethical obligation of physicians to advance the interests of their patients. These contracts also violate the ethical guidelines established by the Council, which demand the disclosure of all treatment options regardless of limitations imposed by plan coverage.

Other restrictive clauses are more specific, designating a particular pathway through which information must pass before reaching patients. Although the language may vary from contract to contract, the system described generally involves a process by which treatment proposals are circulated through some form of utilization review before they are presented to the patient. In effect, physicians who are bound by these contracts require authorization to present treatment options to patients. It stands to reason that because this process exists, the contracting plan anticipates that some proposals will not be authorized and thus not presented. As a result, under this system patients may not be given all the available treatment options from which to choose the best therapeutic course. This failure to disclose all legitimate therapies is paternalistic, deceptive, and cannot be excused by limitations in coverage. Furthermore, standards of informed consent are impossible to uphold when patients are not given information outlining all the possible treatments.

A final category of restrictive clauses prevents physicians from discussing various plan operations including structures of financial reimbursement and utilization review procedures. The Council previously concluded that systems of reimbursement that include incentives to limit care must be disclosed to patients.[2] In general, the financial structure of a plan as well as the mechanism of its quality assurance program could impact the care a patient receives and should therefore be disclosed by the plan prior to enrollment and clarified by the physician thereafter. The exact level of reimbursement, however, constitutes proprietary information and does not need to be disclosed to patients.

Ethical Concerns Common to Clauses Restricting Communication

The practice of medicine is dependent upon the capacity of patients to trust their physicians. Simply stated, patients cannot fully trust a physician who has a contractual obligation to conceal relevant information. Furthermore, society cannot trust that the medical profession is dedicated to the interests of each individual patient when some physicians are bound to agreements that preclude the fulfillment of even the basic duty of disclosure. Public perception often unfairly projects the constraints of some plans onto all managed care providers and ultimately onto all providers. Consequently, even if the majority of physicians have not signed contracts containing disclosure restrictions, the damage to the public trust rendered by the conflicting obligations of the remaining minority will be profound. The danger of undermining society's confidence in medicine demands the profession's vigorous opposition to these clauses and their inappropriate restrictions.

In addition to the loss of public trust resulting from the enforcement of these contracts, the direct impact of these clauses on those patients enrolled in plans employing restrictions on disclosure must be considered. For instance, patients under the care of physicians whose contractual obligations prevent complete disclosure may follow recommendations for treatment without hearing of other, potentially more effective, options. Even if the plan would not cover other options, it is the right of the patient to seek or utilize alternative means to fund therapies outside of the plan. Perhaps more significantly, these patients will surrender unknowingly their right to fully informed consent and will place their faith in a patient-physician relationship formed and maintained under false pretenses. The importance of maintaining the openness and honesty that form the basis of the patient-physician relationship cannot be overstated and requires the rejection of contract clauses which strike at the very heart of that relationship.

Conclusion

The Council has previously written, "The duty of patient advocacy is a fundamental element of the physician-patient relationship that should not be altered by the system of health care delivery in which physicians practice. Physicians must continue to place the interests of their patients first."[2] Whatever the societal implications of "gag clauses" may be, their immediate impact on the ability of physicians to provide information to their patients and to act effectively as a patient advocate is deeply disturbing. Violations of individual and public trust in the profession of medicine are detrimental to the health of society and must be resisted. To facilitate the continued practice of ethical medicine, the Council recommends the following:

1. Managed care organizations have the right to protect proprietary information as long as such protection does not inhibit physicians from disclosing relevant information to patients. Contract clauses which could be applied to prevent physicians from raising or discussing matters relevant to patients' medical care should be removed to safeguard the health of plan subscribers.

2. The right of patients to be informed of all pertinent medical information must be reaffirmed by the medical profession, and individual physicians must continue to uphold their ethical obligation to disclose such information.

3. Physicians should review their contracts carefully to ensure that there is no possibility that the health of their patients will be jeopardized in any way by clauses that inhibit their ability to fulfill their ethical obligations.

Report of the Council on Ethical and Judicial Affairs of the American Medical Association.
June 1996.

Endnotes

1. Council on Ethical and Judicial Affairs, American Medical Association. Fundamental Elements of the Patient-Physician Relationship. *Code of Medical Ethics: Current Opinions with Annotations.* Chicago: American Medical Association: 1994.

2. Council on Ethical and Judicial Affairs, American Medical Association. Ethical Issues in Managed Care. *JAMA.* 273;4:330-335.

Ethical Issues in Negotiating Discounts for Specialty Care

Resolution 9 was introduced by the New England delegation and referred through the Board of Trustees to the Council on Ethical and Judicial Affairs at the 1994 Interim Meeting. This resolution questioned the ethical nature of negotiating discounts between individual specialists and primary care physicians within a system of global capitation. Resolution 9 was motivated by accounts of certain primary care physicians who were abusing their position as a source of referrals to secure discounts from individual specialists. Specifically, these primary care physician were attempting to secure discounts from individual specialists for their globally capitated patients by making such discounts a condition for referring any patients, including those not in the capitated plan. In response to these reports, the Council presents the following ethical analysis of the behavior that served as the impetus for this resolution.

Background

One practice that many managed care organizations have relied upon to reduce costs is restricting referrals for specialist care to a limited panel of specialty physicians who have agreed to a fee schedule established by the plan. This offers potential subscribers the option of accepting restrictions on choice of specialists in exchange for other coverage benefits or lower premiums. These restrictions are acceptable if the patient is informed and agrees to the terms of the plan. It is important to note, however, that many patients and employers have chosen to avoid the restrictions imposed by a closed panel of physicians by selecting coverage that applies to the services of any physician.

Negotiation of Discounts

The proliferation of managed care has placed many primary care physicians in the role of case manager for enormous numbers of patients. These physicians are responsible for recognizing which referral restrictions apply to which patients according to the benefits of different insurance plans. Because of the rigid system of referrals found in many managed care organizations, they are also the source of many referrals for the specialists involved in the plan. This role affords the primary care physician a degree of leverage corresponding to his or her control over the direction of patient referrals. While the vast majority of primary care physicians would never abuse their position as the coordinators of specialist care, episodes such as those described at the outset of this report indicate that certain physician have chosen to exploit their influence on patient referrals to exact a discount for specialist care.

The intent of primary care physicians who use their ability to refer as a tool for lowering the cost of specialist care may be to benefit capitated patients by providing more services on the same budget. However, regardless of the motivation for such restrictions, primary care physicians who threaten to withhold all referrals for financial reasons inappropriately restrict the choices of their non-capitated patients, in effect forcing them to accept precisely those limitations they chose to avoid in subscribing to an alternative insurance plan. Patients who purchased coverage on the understanding that their choices would not be further limited cannot be denied access to a particular specialist because of financial negotiations between contracting physicians.

Conclusion

Patients are entitled to all benefits outlined in their insurance plan. Therefore, it is unethical for a referring physician to restrict the referral options of patients who have chosen a plan that provides for access to an unlimited or broad selection of specialist physicians. It is also unethical to base the referral of these patients on a discount for the capitated patients in a primary care physician's practice.

Negotiating discounts for specialty care within a globally capitated plan may raise additional ethical questions which can be answered sufficiently only within the context of a larger report examining global capitation in general. The Council intends to provide such a report in the future.[1]

Report of the Council on Ethical and Judicial Affairs of the American Medical Association.
June 1996.

Endnote

1. Council on Ethical and Judicial Affairs, American Medical Association. The Ethical Issues of Capitation. In: *Proceedings of the House of Delegates of the American Medical Association:* 146th Annual Meeting. Chicago: American Medical Association; 1997:268-273.

The Ethical Implications of Capitation

The systems through which physicians are reimbursed for their services have grown varied and complex. To date, discussion of the actual impact of these changes on the quality of patient care has been limited by a lack of data. However, there is much to be gained from discourse within the profession concerning the potential effects these systems may have. At the Annual Meeting in 1996, the House of Delegates recognized the need for this discourse and adopted Resolution 5, which recommended that:

1. The American Medical Association study the ethical aspects of capitation and its impact on both physicians and their patients; and that

2. These ethical concerns and issues be reviewed by the Council on Ethical and Judicial Affairs.

With the intent of responding to this resolution and of contributing to the necessary discussion of capitation, the Council presents the following report.

Capitation and Financial Incentives

It is crucial to distinguish pure capitation arrangements from other financial incentives as they are traditionally defined. Financial incentives target the monetary interests of physicians and are designed to use the pressure of potential income variations to encourage certain behaviors. Capitation, on the other hand, is defined simply as the payment of a fixed sum per patient per unit time. If capitated payments are given to individual physicians, the physician's salary will be derived from what remains of the capitated pool, and an inherent financial incentive will be created that could affect the provision of care. Other capitated plans, however, provide payments to a group of physicians whose personal incomes are in turn provided through a wide variety of payment systems ranging from salary to bonuses to fee-for-service. In these plans, the immediate parallels between capitation and other, more direct financial incentives are not so clearly established.

Regardless of how the physician is personally reimbursed, the capitated sum is applied to cover the costs incurred in providing a pre-determined set of services to the pool of capitated patients. Physicians may be expected to apply capitated funds to cover only their own services, or as in the case of some primary care physicians, the pool may also be used to cover the provision of outside laboratory tests, specialty care, hospital stays, and ancillary services. Individual physician income may at least partially be attached to the capitated pool through additional financial incentives, such as bonuses or withholds. An analysis of the ethical merits and conflicts associated with such direct incentives is presented in a different Council report.[1] This report intends to address only the ethical implications of providing care for patients under a fixed budget without attempting to analyze the multifarious reimbursement systems that could be applied as a subset of capitation to influence physician behavior.

Capitation has many of the defining characteristics of other financial incentives. By providing a fixed budget with which to treat patients, physicians are motivated to minimize costs because of the possibility that patients could conceivably find themselves without the resources to obtain treatment if the pool is not managed effectively. Additionally, physicians who practice as a part of a group under capitation typically experience significant pressure to stay within the allotted budget from colleagues who share the resource pool and from insurance companies, employers, and other third-party payers. Although it is not clear whether physicians are motivated to be cost-conscious and efficient by the concerns of colleagues, payors, or patients, it seems clear that capitation successfully shifts the mentality of practicing physicians.[2,3,4,5]

Analysis of the Physician's Role Under Capitation

Although operating under a fixed budget does not necessarily introduce the clinician's personal income into the patient-physician relationship, it can alter the role of the physician. Medicine has long held that the primary obligation of physicians is to advocate for the interests of each individual patient. In a capitated environment, however, patients covered by the same pool have overlapping interests, and explicitly tying the care of multiple patients to a single, limited funding source bestows upon the physician an additional obligation to consider the potential depletion of that resource when making treatment decisions. The extent to which these duties are in conflict is dependent upon the strength of each component obligation. Physicians practicing under capitation have an individual responsibility to maintain the resource pool, and the degree of pressure they experience to act on that responsibility is inversely related to the number of physicians in the capitated plan. Very small plans therefore make physicians more acutely aware of their responsibility to the capitated pool, which may in turn create conflicts with their primary obligation to individual patient care.

Even in large plans, physicians practicing under capitation are encouraged to consider the costs to the plan of different treatment options. It is entirely appropriate for physicians to feel some obligation to safeguard broader health care resources; indeed such an obligation has existed for decades.[6] Adopting dual roles is only cause for concern when the roles are given equal or nearly equal status and the primacy of individual patient care is threatened.

The Physician as Insurer

When discussing capitation, it is useful to note some of the parallels between physicians under capitation and insurers. While the analogy is by no means perfect, some comparisons are helpful. Insurers receive, in the form of a premium, a fixed sum from each member of the covered population. With that sum, they are responsible for paying all legitimate claims in order to fulfill the guarantee of protection implied under the term "insurance." Their duty to their subscribers, therefore, is to manage a global budget against shortfalls. Fulfilling this duty requires that they judge individual claims to determine if they in fact meet criteria for coverage. It also requires that they examine each claim in light of its potential impact on the system's ability to pay future claims. All the descriptions to this point could equally describe the position of physicians practicing under capitation.

Perhaps the primary function of insurers can best be described as making broad-level decisions about plan resource allocation. Recognizing that decisions about the application of limited medical resources may be appropriate, the Council has previously stipulated that any allocation decisions that will affect patient access to care must be decided on a broad (ideally societal) level.[7] Given their unique knowledge of what constitutes acceptable levels of health care, the input of physicians into these global decisions is crucial. It is therefore appropriate for large groups of physicians who accept capitated payments together to take an active role in assessing which services will be covered under their capitated resource. It is imperative, however, that such determinations be disclosed to patients prior to their enrollment in the plan.

As physicians under capitation assume many of the roles traditionally held by insurers, however, these decisions could be brought to the bedside. The uncertainties of clinical practice place inherent limits on the degree of precision specific rules for coverage can be expected to attain, and it is tempting to place the burden of allocating resources on the shoulders of individual physicians. This shift in responsibility can be achieved by capitating single physicians or small groups of physicians and allowing them to establish rules of resource utilization. The Council has previously opposed this form of allocation because it depends upon variable factors in an individual's practice and may lead to standards of provision that are not consistent across different physician practices.[7] Furthermore, because these decisions are based in part on the resource use of a relatively small group of patients, fluctuations in clinical practice may result in standards that are not even consistent within one physician's practice across different time periods.

Implications for Patient Care

The effect on patient care of the physician's role as it is defined under capitation ultimately hinges upon the availability of funds to provide treatment. The adequacy of plan resources is affected by a number of factors. First, the efficiency of a physician's practice can impact the availability of resources. By reducing overhead or any unnecessary services, physicians can increase the effective size of the capitated pool.

A second factor is the rate of capitated payment. A capitation rate that is insufficient to fund all necessary care even under circumstances of ideal efficiency could adversely affect the care available to plan patients. Some have argued that setting the capitation rate too low will impact quality and therefore detract from the payor's ability to compete in the medical marketplace. In other words, quality control and patient protection will be provided by market forces. Additionally, it has been argued that medical malpractice claims and liability suits will provide a check against deterioration in the quality of care. The level of protection these safeguards can provide is highly debatable, not least because quality is so hard to assess by any objective available measure. That point notwithstanding, it seems that liability and market forces are tools better suited to preventing a slide below minimal levels of care than to upholding the standards of optimal care.

Regardless of how effective liability and free-market economics may be in protecting patients, the fact remains that as determinants of the capitation rate these issues largely miss the point. Capitation is a means to reduce costs. Its value to the health care system, however, is linked only to its ability to eliminate unnecessary and wasteful practices. In keeping with this goal, the rate of capitation should be determined by the identifiable needs of the covered patients and not by market trends or the probability of legal action. It is difficult for payment rates based on either purely economic or legal premises to reflect the appropriate goals and aims of the profession, including the provision of necessary care and the preservation of ethical practice.

Admittedly, basing capitation payments on a determination of necessary services is difficult given the general lack of consensus even among physicians as to what constitutes optimal care. Debate between professionals concerning specific treatments has long existed and recent data suggest that there are broad differences in practice patterns across geographic areas.[8] An inadequate supply of definitive outcomes data further complicates attempts to define necessary care for a given population, to say nothing of assessing the appropriate cost of that care. However, even an estimate based on available information is superior to a figure that does not attempt to incorporate the nuances of varying levels of care.

It is imperative that the capitation rate reflect the medical needs of plan patients, because a pool that is insufficient to cover necessary care can lead to serious ethical conflicts for the physician. The most obvious of these conflicts arises between patients. If the financial resources are inadequate to the task of providing all necessary care, the physician has no choice but to prioritize individual patients on the basis of relative need. There are a number of implications associated with this process. First, and perhaps most troubling, some patients may be denied care that could be of material benefit. For instance, cases of marginal or discretionary need may be targeted for refusal of treatment, or less costly and less effective treatments may be substituted for more expensive but more effective interventions. As marginal need may become too liberally defined under financial constraints, additional necessary care may be denied.

A second concern raised by inadequate capitation rates is that confidence among patients that the physician is in a position to advocate for their individual needs may be severely undermined. Patients engage in treatment relationships on the assumption that physicians act as advocates for individuals. They cannot assume that all requested treatments will be paid for or even provided, but they can rely upon their physicians to act in a manner that is responsive to their particular needs. Encouraging a physician to deny or alter care for one patient on the basis of the competing needs of another patient will have significant and deleterious effects on the trust that lies at the core of the patient-physician relationship.

Mitigating Ethical Concerns at the Level of a Capitated Plan

Because the capitation rate is so pivotal in the ethical analysis of the system, the factors that should be considered when evaluating the size of a capitated payment need to be stated. First, the individual medical needs of enrolled patients should be assessed and accommodated in the capitated plan. This can be accomplished in a number of ways. For example, capitated payments made to each physician can be adjusted according to the general characteristics (age, gender, existing chronic conditions) of the patients represented in his or her practice. In this way, physicians with a disproportionate number of sick patients will be given a slightly larger capitated pool from which to provide appropriate care. Even more simply, the expenses generated by a similar patient population in previous years can be used as a benchmark to establish a capitated rate that will facilitate the provision of necessary care.

The uncertainties of clinical practice preclude the establishment of exact capitation figures, and while medical factors and parameters of necessary care

are indispensable to the process of setting capitation rates, they can lead to only a close approximation of probable costs. These estimates are superior to rates set on the basis of market economics but still result in risks that the pool will be inadequate to provide all required care. For this reason, additional means to protect patients in a capitated system from the potential effects of budgetary shortfalls need to be considered. For instance, the size of the plan can mitigate or prevent fluctuations in costs that will lead to unpredicted but necessary rationing on the part of the physician. The laws of probability dictate that the expenses incurred by a very large patient population over an extended period of time will consistently approximate a definable average. The Health Care Financing Administration has estimated that the expenses incurred by patient populations in excess of 25,000 members do not vary significantly from year to year.[9] It seems then that spreading financial risk by capitating large pools of patients will reduce variations in the available budget and therefore prevent physicians from having to base their treatment decisions on unforeseen or potential budgetary crises. This approach also improves the ability of plans to predict annual expenses and to set the rate of capitation according to the foreseeable use of resources.

Increasing the number of physicians who are capitated as a group will have a similar effect on the level of financial risk as increasing the size of the patient pool. By providing capitated funds to a large physician group, the effect of any single treatment decision on the pool of resources is diluted, thereby reducing the incentive to consider potentially competing interests of other patients while providing treatment to individuals. Sharing a capitated pool over a group also promotes the mutual assumption of responsibility for treatment decisions, which in turn promotes peer review between group physicians and reduces the element of individual responsibility for allocation decisions.

The time over which capitation rates are calculated will also affect the accuracy of predicted use and will therefore affect the physician's perception of the impact individual clinical decisions may have on the available budget. Increasing the time period over which resource use is measured greatly increases the probability that excessive costs will be counterbalanced by periods of underutilization. This dissipates the immediacy of the cause and effect relationship between one clinical treatment and the ability to provide other interventions in the future.

Even under ideal circumstances, the capitated physician runs the risk that a small number of patients could require a level of care sufficiently extreme to create a conflict with the interests of other patients covered through the same pool of capitated funds. Most plans and physicians recognize the need for protection against such an occurrence and have provided some form of stop-loss plan. Once a set spending limit is reached, these plans pay the vast majority of costs incurred in treating individual patients. The need for these provisions is underscored by the fact that even the possibility of a catastrophic case could seem sufficiently pervasive to encourage physicians to treat their patients too conservatively in order to preserve funds against such an event. It could also lead plans to identify those patients likely to require such catastrophic care and to discourage or prevent their inclusion in a capitated pool. As neither of these options is acceptable, protection against excessive losses resulting from the treatment of a single patient must be implemented.

Mitigating Ethical Concerns on the Level of the Physician

Even with safeguards, physicians have an obligation to determine if the rate of payment is sufficient to provide all necessary care. In previous reports, the Council has established an obligation on the part of physicians to appeal denials of coverage for necessary treatments. Capitated physicians have a corresponding responsibility to appeal for a larger budget if established payments are inadequate to the task of providing care. Similarly, physicians have an obligation to ensure that the pool for which capitated payments apply is sufficiently large to compensate for unpredictable variations in the cost of providing services. As a final protection, physicians should be covered through some form of stop-loss plan.

Assessing the rate of capitation as an individual physician is clearly a difficult task. As a general rule, however, payment systems can be judged in part on the basis of whether or not they are appropriate to discuss with patients. Patients have a right to all information that may impact on the care they receive, including the reimbursement plan under which that care is delivered.

Physicians should avoid arrangements that cannot be justified to patients and therefore cannot be disclosed without negatively affecting the patient-physician relationship.

Conclusion

Appropriately constructed, capitation can be applied to reduce the costs of health care and further the interests of patients, physicians and the health care system in general. Capitation encourages physicians to act on their obligation to the health of more global populations through increased efficiency and attention to necessary allocation decisions. Even under ideal circumstances, however, providing physicians with a fixed budget not only encourages attention to broader obligations, but also requires physicians to recognize and consider potential conflicts that may exist between patients in the course of clinical care. While it is difficult for capitated physicians to ignore the competing demands of the larger group, they must continue to fulfill their primary obligation to act as single-minded advocates for the needs of each individual patient.

If not carefully constructed, systems of capitation can create conflicts that can in turn impact patient care. If physicians have insufficient funds available to provide all necessary care, plan patients will be placed in competition for plan resources, and the physicians may be forced to evaluate patient need on a relative scale with the intent of minimizing expenditures rather than maximizing quality of care. There is also the possibility that inappropriately designed systems may result in discrimination against the sick. The potential for these conflicts to arise is influenced by a number of factors, including the rate of capitation, the size of the patient pool covered by capitated payments, the size of the physician group for whom the pool applies, and the time period over which capitated rates are calculated.

Recommendations

The Council recognizes that the application of capitation to physicians' practices can result in the provision of cost-effective, quality medical care. It is important to note, however, that the potential for conflict exists under such systems. In an effort to minimize these conflicts and to ensure that capitation is applied in a manner consistent with the interests of patients, the Council recommends the following:

1. Physicians have an obligation to evaluate a health plan's capitation payments prior to contracting with that plan to ensure that the quality of

patient care is not threatened by inadequate rates of capitation. Capitation payments should be calculated primarily on relevant medical factors, available outcomes data, the costs associated with involved providers, and consensus oriented standards of necessary care. Furthermore, the predictable costs resulting from existing conditions of enrolled patients should be considered when determining the rate of capitation. Different populations of patients have different medical needs and the cost s associated with those needs should be reflected in the per member per month payment. Physicians should seek agreements with plans that provide sufficient financial resources for all necessary care and should refuse to sign agreements that fail in this regard.

2. Physicians must not assume inordinate levels of financial risk and should therefore consider a number of factors when deciding whether or not to sign a provider agreement. The size of the plan and the time period over which the rate is figured should be considered by physicians evaluating a plan as well as in determinations of the per member per month payment. The capitation rate for large plans can be calculated more accurately than for smaller plans because of the mitigating influence of probability and the behavior of large systems. Similarly, length of time will influence the predictability of patient expenditures and should be considered accordingly. Capitation rates calculated for large plans over an extended period of time are able to be more accurate and are therefore preferable to those calculated for small groups over a short time period.

3. Stop-loss plans should be in effect to prevent the potential of catastrophic expenses from influencing physician behavior. Physicians should ensure that such arrangements are finalized prior to signing an agreement to provide services in a health plan.

4. Physicians must be prepared to discuss with patients any financial arrangements which could impact patient care. Physicians should avoid reimbursement systems that cannot be disclosed to patients without negatively affecting the patient-physician relationship.

Report of the Council on Ethical and Judicial Affairs of the American Medical Association.
June 1997.

Endnotes

1. Council on Ethical and Judicial Affairs, American Medical Association. Financial Incentives and the Practice of Medicine. In: *Proceedings of the House of Delegates of the American Medical Association: 51st Interim Meeting*. Chicago: American Medical Association; 1997.

2. Epstein AM, Begg CV, and McNeil, BJ. The Use of Ambulatory Testing in Prepaid and Fee-For-Service Group Practices. *N Engl J Med.* 1986;312:1089-1094.

3. Hillman, AL, Pauly MV, and Kerstein JJ. How do Financial Incentives Affect Physicians' Clinical Decisions and the Financial Performance of Health Maintenance Organizations? *N Engl J Med.* 1989;321:86-92.

4. Clancy CM, Hillner BE. Physicians as Gatekeepers: The Impact of Financial Incentives. *Arch of Intern Med.* 1989;149:917-920.

5. Kosecoff, et al. Prospective Payment System and Impairment at Discharge. *JAMA.* 1990;264:1980-1983.

6. See Principle Vll, AMA Principles of Medical Ethics. In: *Code of Medical Ethics: Current Opinions with Annotations.* Chicago: American Medical Association; 1996.

7. Council on Ethical and Judicial Affairs, American Medical Association. Ethical Issues in Managed Care. *JAMA.* 1995;273:330-335.

8. Wennberg, JE et al. *The Dartmouth Atlas of Health Care.* American Hospital Publishing: 1996.

9. See 42 CFR ¤ 4 1 7.479(h)(1)(v) as published at 61 Fed. Reg. 69,049-69,050.

Financial Incentives and the Practice of Medicine

Several past Council reports and opinions have addressed, directly or indirectly, the ethical implications of practicing medicine in an environment that provides financial rewards and penalties to physicians.[1] The House of Delegates has also examined the issues surrounding financial incentives, and has produced a number of policy statements relating generally to the application of monetary inducements to the practice of medicine.[2] Despite the wide variety of issues these past statements address, they are all based on a fundamental appreciation of the patient-physician relationship and the role of the profession in advocating for the medical needs of each patient. Maintaining a focus on this ethical foundation is increasingly important as the nation's health care system continues to evolve and the methods of physician reimbursement continue to change. Although it is impossible to provide a discrete ethical analysis of each model of physician reimbursement, the Council presents this report in an effort to highlight the fundamental ethical concerns of any health care payment regime.

Background

There are numerous types of financial incentives, including bonuses attached to specific patterns of practice or utilization goals, payments made out of a pool of withheld funds used to cover the cost of referral services, and fee-for-service payments. The many forms and combinations of incentive payments are often divided into two categories according to the "direction" in which they encourage physicians to move along the spectrum of utilization. This simple system distinguishes between incentives to provide care and incentives to limit resource use. For example, paying physicians on a fee-for-service basis provides an inducement to provide more services. On the other hand, paying physicians a portion of whatever balance remains in a pool of funds used first to cover referral services strongly encourages physicians to reduce utilization.

Although the system of categorization described above can be a useful model for discussion, it has important shortcomings. The choice of "direction" as the defining characteristic of a particular incentive is often not value-neutral. It is often assumed that providing more care is preferable to providing less, and that incentives to limit care are necessarily worse than those that encourage resource utilization. This assumption persists, despite the lack of conclusive data linking different incentives to reductions in quality of care. Identifying the "direction" of an incentive also does little to reflect the underlying goal or goals of a particular payment regime, focusing instead exclusively on levels of utilization. Finally, such a system of labeling incentives has no category for those incentives that are not directly related to providing or limiting services, such as incentives that target improvements in quality and patient satisfaction.

This report resists separating incentive plans into these two categories. It attempts, instead, to find the elements common to all, and to provide general guidance on the ethical implications of introducing the financial interest of the physician into the treatment relationship. Having established the ethical parameters governing the universe of incentives, it will be possible to provide more specific guidelines to ensure that the goals of the profession are protected and in fact actualized.

One element common to different financial incentive plans is that they encourage specific behaviors by penalizing or rewarding physicians on the basis of their patterns of clinical practice. Although fee-for-service medicine was not introduced as an explicit incentive, several studies have shown that providing a financial return for each service rendered can have an impact on the decision-making process of some physicians.[3,4,5] Noting the effectiveness of incentives at modifying clinical behavior, managed care organizations have developed a wide variety of payment mechanisms that target either specific practices or general patterns of care in an effort to reduce the cost of providing care to plan patients.

Financial incentive plans also share the same general hazards. Regardless of the specific behavior targeted for a monetary inducement, the potential exists to create a conflict of interest involving the needs of the patient and the personal financial interests of the treating physician. For instance, a sufficiently large bonus tied to reducing the length of hospital stays could force a physician to choose between a substantial portion of his or her income and potentially beneficial care for patients. Although the ethic of the profession demands that physicians provide their patients with all necessary care regardless of the personal reward or penalty involved,[6] the conflict becomes particularly acute in cases of marginal need, or when the benefits of treatment are uncertain. Fee-for-service medicine creates a similar conflict, except that the physician is inclined by his or her financial interests to provide care that is only marginally indicated.

Although medicine has a long tradition requiring physicians to resolve these conflicts to the benefit of the patient, avoiding or minimizing these conflicts is important, both to the patient's perception of clinical objectivity and to the physician's ability to practice medicine as an advocate for the patient. It is appropriate and important, therefore, for the profession to establish the goals upon which incentive plans should be based and to provide basic parameters that protect the system of fundamental values governing physician behavior.

Goals for the Application of Incentives

The most fundamental goal of the medical profession is to provide for the health of patients. Applied broadly, this objective encompasses a commitment to safeguard the public health through the provision of quality, cost-effective care and to extend access to adequate health care to every individual.[7] Applied in the context of clinical care, this requires physicians to place the health interests of their individual patients before all other concerns, and to facilitate access to all necessary treatments. Financial incentives should be designed around this principle and ultimately judged according to their success or failure at fostering improvements in patient care.

Incentives should also be judged according to the extent to which they foster the treatment relationship between patient and physician by allowing physicians to assume their role as advocates for the health of individual patients. Physicians should never be discouraged by incentives from fulfilling their obligations to disclose all treatment options, to appeal any denials of coverage for necessary care, to make referrals on the basis of individual patient needs, and to provide to each patient those treatments which they believe be of material benefit. Individual patients do not behave according to statistics, and physicians must have the freedom to recognize and to accommodate the specific medical, financial, and psychosocial needs of the individuals in their practices.

Potential Benefits of Employing Financial Incentives

One of the strongest potential benefits financial incentives can provide is a reduction of waste in the application of medical resources, thereby effectively increasing the pool of resources for care. Fee-for-service medicine provides no incentive for physicians to economize use, and abuses of that system are manifest in cases of overutilization. Incentives can be applied to eliminate inefficiencies and defensive practices that may lead to artificial inflation of health care costs. Such incentives can be tailored to encourage the conservative but appropriate provision of medical care, thus maximizing the benefit gained from limited resources. For example, assuming appropriate utilization could be established by objective means, bonuses could be paid to physicians on the basis of their success at applying resources in an effective and efficient manner.

Applying incentives to specific patterns of care allows health plans to encourage a shift in practice towards preventive medicine and ambulatory care. Not only can such a shift produce cost savings, it can encourage physicians to become more involved in the health-related lifestyle choices of their patients. Ultimately, it can also improve the long-term health of patients. Additionally, incentives can be used to reward the integration and coordination of services, benefiting patients by providing more convenient access to care at a variety of levels.

A final advantage afforded by many incentive programs is the increased attention paid on a system level to patient satisfaction. Many managed care entities tie bonuses or reimbursement to patient surveys critiquing the performance of physicians and the managed care organization itself. Such plans encourage physicians to provide quality care and give patients the opportunity to voice any concerns they have regarding the level or type of care available through their plan.

Potential Risks Associated With Financial Incentives

Financial incentives operate by involving the personal interests of the physician in the therapeutic relationship. Physicians have a long-established obligation to put the interests of patients before all others, and in the majority of treatment circumstances, the appropriate manifestation of this obligation is clear. No physician can justify denying a patient absolutely necessary care or providing clearly unnecessary care, regardless of the incentive involved. However, there are certainly cases in which multiple treatment options exist, and in which the best among them is not abundantly clear. The physician must then exercise his or her judgment and weigh the probabilities of benefit against potential harms, taking into consideration factors including efficacy and cost in an effort to identify the treatment (or lack of treatment) most likely to benefit the patient.

The effect of financial incentives is felt most acutely in situations such as this, when the clinical imperfections of medicine become apparent and the physician is called upon to render an objective analysis of several complex considerations. It is exceedingly difficult to maintain true objectivity when a monetary reward or penalty is associated with a specific course of action. While this inducement will have little, if any, effect when the best treatment course is clear, its influence will grow as the gap separating different clinical options shrinks and the effects of each become similar. It is not reasonable to expect that all physicians can resist completely the influence of a financial incentive on true borderline cases. It is therefore critical to place limits on financial incentives to ensure that clinical objectivity is protected.

The potential to affect the objectivity of physicians is not the only cause for concern associated with financial incentives. Inducements that are based on the use of resources across physicians' practices compound the conflict between the interests of the physician and those of the patient by introducing conflicts between patients. When physicians are provided with incentives to meet specific levels of utilization, they are encouraged to consider the needs of the individual patient relative to the needs of other patients. For instance, bonuses attached to patterns of reduced use encourage physicians to consider which patients need certain services *most,* rather than simply which patients need certain services. Such an incentive would not, in all likelihood, have any noticeable impact in cases of clear patient need. Again, however, these incentives would have a greater impact on the care offered in cases of potential, but unclear, benefit.

Incentives that encourage physicians to consider the needs of patients in relation to one another could impact the ability of physicians to carry out their fundamental obligation of individual patient advocacy. Whether or not physicians are ever forced by incentives into a form of circumstantial or "bedside" rationing, patients may feel as though they must compete for scarce resources in a forum lacking significant oversight or consistent structure. The essential premise that physicians act wholly in the interests of each individual, constrained only by publicly determined limits on resources, allows patients to trust their physicians. Any incentive plan that challenges or appears to challenge this fundamental notion could have a far-reaching impact on the patient-physician relationship.

Even the appearance of rationing hints at perhaps the most troubling side-effect of incentive programs, namely their potential to disrupt the trust that exists between patients and physicians. No consequence of applying financial incentives would be more destructive to patient care than a widespread degradation of the public trust in the medical profession. While perceived competition between patients for resources could cast doubt on the ability of the treating physician to act as an individual advocate, the simple fact that a physician could stand to reap significant financial gain by providing (or not providing) a specific form of care may raise fundamental questions about the therapeutic relationship. This challenge to the patient's conception of medical practice could arise regardless of the actual effect any given incentive has, or does not have, on the clinical decision-making process.

Disclosure of Financial Incentives

Since the existence of financial incentives alone could impact the patient-physician relationship, developing an appropriate strategy to disclose those incentives is not a straightforward task. Patients have a right to be informed of all factors that could impact their care, including the payment system under which their physician practices. Disclosure is also necessary because the sense of betrayal and suspicion that would result from the independent discovery of a system capable of affecting clinical judgment would far outweigh the impact of full disclosure.

A much more difficult question to answer than whether or not to disclose incentives is where the responsibility for providing such information lies. A compelling argument can be made for disclosure prior to enrollment in a health plan, as the structure of financial inducements could influence the patient's decision to purchase a specific form of coverage.[8] However, if disclosure of the nature of financial arrangements between payer and physician does not occur at the level of the payer, some obligation exists on the part of the physician to provide that information.

Effects of Financial Incentives on the Profession

The biggest concern associated with financial incentives is the conflict of interest they generate and the possible impact of that conflict on clinical objectivity and patient care. However, the ramifications of monetary inducements are by no means limited to the health of patients; they extend to physicians' perceptions of the profession and their role in caring for patients. The reaction of many physicians to the increasingly prevalent tension between personal economic interests and the therapeutic relationship has been one of discontent. In many ways, the application of financial incentives to reduce or limit utilization has changed the manner in which physicians are being asked to treat patients. The bottom line requires constant attention, breeding resentment towards those patients who require the most care and resources. Physicians are implicitly or even explicitly encouraged to shorten office visits and to reduce the use of certain services. Many recognize the inherent conflict of interest created through the use of financial incentives, but feel they have few options available to alleviate that conflict. The effect of this discontent on the patient-physician relationship and ultimately on the practice of medicine is not yet clear, but is cause for some concern.

Another sentiment common among physicians is that many financial incentives are transforming their station in the health care system. Physicians have defined themselves as a profession by their dedication to the principles of ethical practice, their dedication to the individual patient, and their ability to weigh these and other factors in determining the appropriate course of treatment for the sick. In many ways, the increased use and specificity of financial incentives is challenging this definition. The practice of medicine is not an exact science and relies heavily upon the ability of physicians to interpret a number of conditions other than physiological symptoms when recommending treatment. And yet, some financial incentive plans tied directly to average utilization rates encourage physicians to treat in exactly the same way all patients presenting the same or similar symptoms. In this way, many plans attempt to define rigidly what has for years been the purview of professional judgment and expert interpretation of nonquantifiable factors. The end result may be that physicians question their status as professionals in the face of increased micromanagement through utilization review and bonus schedules.

Limiting the Influence of Incentives to Preserve the Goals of the Profession

The Council has long recognized the primacy of patient interests, stating in part, "If a conflict develops between the physician's financial interest and the physician's responsibilities to the patient, the conflict must be resolved to the patient's benefit."[9] This broad statement applies equally to all financial conflicts engendered by incentives. There is also an obligation on the part of the medical profession to protect medical resources against waste and thereby to minimize the costs borne by patients. The intersection of these obligations provides a standard with which to judge the ethical propriety of various incentive plans. Well-designed plans encourage the appropriate use of medical resources without creating conflicts of interest that could impact individual, clinical care. Poorly-designed plans are either ineffective at encouraging efficiency, or intrusive on the independent judgment of patient and physician. In light of this standard, the task before the profession is to provide a framework identifying the factors that influence the degree to which different incentive plans allow physicians to uphold their ethical commitments.

The size of the financial reward or penalty associated with certain practices can help distinguish appropriate from inappropriate incentives. All other factors being equal, a direct correlation exists between the size of a financial inducement and the degree of influence it exercises. Large bonuses are more likely to affect objectivity than smaller ones, and placing a large portion of a physician's income at risk for treatment decisions creates a more substantial conflict of interest than placing a small percentage of potential earnings at risk.

Although the size of the incentive is important, it is not the sole determinant of ethical propriety and often works in conjunction with other factors. For instance, the proximity of an incentive to an individual act is crucial in predicting its eventual influence on services rendered. Proximity is a function of the degree to which physicians can reap personal benefit from individual treatment decisions rather than broader patterns of practice. The closer the proximity of an incentive to individual clinical encounters, the more likely it is to be given undue consideration.

Perhaps the most direct incentive is provided by a system of fee-for-service in which a direct correlation is established between individual service and payment. Unethical conduct under such circumstances can come in a variety of forms, including the provision of unnecessary services, self-referral, and fee-splitting. It is difficult to create systemic limitations which can eliminate these abuses; however, the individual acts themselves are readily identified and proscribed.[10] In addition to prohibiting these specific abuses, the Council has issued guidelines governing the establishment of appropriate fees in an effort to ensure that physicians charge rates commensurate with their skill and training.[11]

The influence on clinical practice of most other forms of financial incentives can be limited by altering the proximity of the incentive to specific clinical encounters. Spreading the risks can dilute incentives and benefits accrued through individual treatment decisions across panels of physicians. Because the savings generated by one individual physician will benefit a group, the amount the individual stands to gain from any single act is dramatically reduced. Likewise, in those situations where personal income is placed at risk, physicians who share that risk stand to lose substantially less potential income as a result of any single clinical decision. In either case, an incentive to practice in accordance with standards of efficiency exists; however, the immediacy of that incentive to individual treatment options is dramatically reduced.

Similar to applying incentives across broad physician groups, the proximity of incentives to single decisions can also be reduced by tying inducements to experience related to a large patient pool. As the laws of probability dictate, larger patient populations are more likely to have stable and predictable health care needs. When considering the care offered to a large number of patients, it becomes clear that expensive or extensive treatments for one patient will be balanced by the relatively minor or non-existent needs of others. Because the physician whose incentive plan applies to a large group can rely upon other cases to balance the needs of even exceptional patients, the freedom to exercise clinical judgment is preserved.

Following the same laws of probability, it becomes clear that incentives attached to utilization can also be limited by calculating patterns of use over longer rather than shorter periods of time. Despite potentially wide variations in individual care, the mean rates of resource consumption more closely approximate a consistent average as the time period over which they are calculated expands. Therefore, lengthening the time frame over which incentive payments are calculated reduces the risk that any one treatment decision will have a significant impact on the physician's financial reward or penalty.

It is important to note that some incentive plans that appear on their face to incentivize treatment patterns rather than individual decisions may in fact create circumstances in which enormous and unintended inducements result. Incentives that are awarded when a discrete point of utilization is achieved may satisfy the requirement to consider the use of resources across broad patterns of care. In some situations, though, they may create untenable conflicts. For instance, a bonus attached to an increased number of patient visits may be awarded in its entirety when the physician reaches a specific number of clinical encounters. As the end of the fiscal period approaches, if the physician is within striking distance of that goal, an enormous incentive is created to see enough patients to realize what might be a substantial bonus.

Consider the case of a physician who stands to be awarded a $15,000 bonus if he can conduct 8,000 patient visits in a year. If, on the other hand, he conducts 7,999 visits, he receives nothing. In the last week of the year, $15,000 may ride on his ability to see 200 patients and a coercive incentive is established. In general, it is necessary to guard against the possibility that an incentive intended for annual or broadly calculated patterns could effectively ride on a much smaller number of individual cases. Consequently, incentives that are established on a continuum of utilization rather than a system of bracketed cutoff points will be more likely to prevent potentially severe conflicts of interest.

Even with safeguards in place, catastrophic care for a single patient can in many instances have a significant impact on the incentive payment that a physician receives. It is important, therefore, to provide some further protection from the potentially significant impact any treatment for a single patient could have on the income of a physician. The best means to achieve this protection is through the provision of a stop-loss plan. When the costs of treatment for a single patient climb above a fixed level, an insurance policy or an overflow pool of funds pays the majority of the balance. This allows physicians to recommend and provide treatment that would otherwise deplete a pool of withheld money or skew the appearance of their utilization rate.

A final means through which the potentially negative effects of financial incentives can be avoided is to include among other specific mechanism rewards and penalties tied to quality measures. This will reinforce the importance of establishing efficient but effective practice patterns. It also provides a simple check against any movement to view reductions in utilization, rather than the provision of optimal care, as the primary goal.

Conclusion

The purpose of incentive plans is to motivate physicians to eliminate waste and to provide optimal levels of care. The specific mechanisms used to achieve this goal should therefore be tailored in accordance with predictions of utilization dictated by medical necessity rather than by market economics and a plan's competitive standing. Physicians should not be offered monetary incentives that are designed to reduce costs below levels compatible with the provision of all necessary care. Such inducements introduce conflicts of interest that encroach upon the therapeutic relationship and threaten individual and public trust in the profession. To protect against such eventualities, the health needs of each patient, and the ability of physicians to act as individual advocates, must remain the principal considerations of any reimbursement plan.

Recommendations

In order to achieve the necessary goals of patient care and to protect the role of physicians as advocates for individual patient needs, the Council recommends the following:

1. Although physicians have an obligation to consider the needs of broader patient populations within the context of the physician-patient relationship, their first duty must be to the individual patient. This obligation must override considerations of the reimbursement mechanism or specific financial incentives applied to a physician's clinical practice.

2. Physicians, individually or through their representatives, should evaluate the financial incentives associated with participation in a health plan before contracting with that plan. The purpose of the evaluation is to ensure that quality of patient care is not compromised by unrealistic expectations for utilization or by placing that physician's payments for care at excessive risk. In the process of making judgments about the ethical propriety of such reimbursement systems, physicians should refer to the following general guidelines:

(a) Monetary incentives may be judged in part on the basis of their size. Large incentives may create conflicts of interest that can in turn compromise clinical objectivity. While an obligation has been established to resolve financial conflicts of interest to the benefit of patients, it is important to recognize that sufficiently large incentives can create an untenable position for physicians.

(b) The proximity of large financial incentives to individual treatment decisions should be limited in order to prevent physicians' personal financial concerns from creating a conflict with their role as individual patient advocates. When the proximity of incentives cannot be mitigated, as in the case of fee-for-service payments, physicians must behave in accordance with prior Council recommendations limiting the potential for abuse. This includes the Council's prohibitions on fee-splitting arrangements, the provision of unnecessary services, unreasonable fees, and self-referral. For incentives that can be distanced from clinical decisions, the following factors should be considered in order to evaluate the correlation between individual act and monetary reward or penalty.

i. In general, incentives should be applied across broad physician groups. This dilutes the effect any one physician can have on his or her financial situation through clinical recommendations, thus allowing physicians to provide those services they feel are necessary in each case. Simultaneously, however, physicians are encouraged by the incentive to practice efficiently.

ii. The size of the patient pool considered in calculations of incentive payments will affect the proximity of financial motivations to individual treatment decisions. The laws of probability dictate that in large populations of patients, the overall level of utilization remains relatively stable and predictable. Physicians practicing in plans with large numbers of patients in a risk pool therefore have greater freedom to provide the care they feel is necessary based on the likelihood that the needs of other plan patients will balance out decisions to provide extensive care.

iii. The time period over which incentives are determined should be long enough to accommodate fluctuations in utilization resulting from the random distribution of patients and illnesses. For example, basing incentive payments on an annual analysis of resource utilization is preferable to basing them on monthly review.

iv. Financial rewards or penalties that are triggered by specific points of utilization may create enormous incentives as a physician's practice approaches the established level. Incentives should therefore be calculated on a continuum of utilization rather than a bracketed system with tiers of widely varied bonuses or penalties.

v. A stop-loss plan should be in place to prevent the costs of treating a single patient from significantly impacting the reward or penalty offered to a physician.

3. Incentives should be designed to promote efficient practice, but should not be designed to realize cost savings beyond those attainable through efficiency. As a counterbalance to the focus on utilization reduction, incentives should also be based upon measures of quality of care and patient satisfaction.

4. Patients must be informed of financial incentive that could impact the level or type of care they receive. This responsibility should be assumed by the health plan to ensure that patients are aware of such incentives prior to enrollment. Physicians, individually or through their representatives, must be prepared to discuss with patients any financial arrangements that could impact patient care. Physicians should avoid reimbursement systems that cannot be disclosed to patients without negatively affecting the physician-patient relationship.

Report of the Council on Ethical and Judicial Affairs of the American Medical Association.
December 1997.

Endnotes

1. Council on Ethical and Judicial Affairs, American Medical Association. Opinions 4.01, 4.03, 6.01, 6.02, 6.03, 6.04, 6.05, 6.10, 8.03, 8.031, 8.032, 8.035, 8.06, 8.061, 8.13, 8.132, 8.135, 9.011. In: *Code of Medical Ethics: Current Opinions with Annotations.* Chicago: American Medical Association; 1996.

2. American Medical Association. Policies 140.978, 285, 982. In: *American Medical Association Policy Compendium.* Chicago: American Medical Association, 1996.

3. Clancy CM and Hillner, BE. Physicians as Gatekeepers: The Impact of Financial Incentives. *Arch lntern Med.* 1989;149:917-920.

4. Epstein AM, Begg CB, McNeil BJ. The Use of Ambulatory Testing in Prepaid and Fee-For-Service Group Practices. *N Engl J Med.* 1986;314:1089-1094.

5. Hemenway D, et al. Physicians' Responses to Financial Incentives. *N Engl J Med.* 1990;322:1059-1063.

6. Council on Ethical and Judicial Affairs, American Medical Association. Opinion 8.03, 8.13. In: *Code of Medical Ethics: Current Opinions with Annotations.* Chicago: American Medical Association; 1996.

7. Council on Ethical and Judicial Affairs, American Medical Association. Ethical Issues in health cares system reform: The provisions of adequate health care. In: *Code of Medical Ethics: Reports of the Ethical and Judicial Affairs of the American Medical Association,* Vol. V. Chicago: American Medical Association; 1994:195-207.

8. Council on Ethical and Judicial Affairs of the American Medical Association. "Ethical Issues in Managed Care." *JAMA.* 1995;273:330-335.

9. See endnote 6

10. See endnote 1

11. Council on Ethical and Judicial Affairs, American Medical Association. Opinion 6.05. In: *Code of Medical Ethics: Current Opinions with Annotations.* Chicago: American Medical Association; 1996.